The Marriage of the Sun and Moon

Books by Andrew Weil, M.D.

THE NATURAL MIND
A Revolutionary Approach to the Drug Problem

THE MARRIAGE OF THE SUN AND MOON
Dispatches from the Frontiers of Consciousness

FROM CHOCOLATE TO MORPHINE
Everything You Need to Know About
Mind-Altering Drugs (*with Winifred Rosen*)

HEALTH AND HEALING
The Philosophy of Integrative Medicine

NATURAL HEALTH, NATURAL MEDICINE
The Complete Guide to Wellness and
Self-Care for Optimum Health

SPONTANEOUS HEALING
How to Discover and Enhance the
Body's Ability to Maintain and Heal Itself

EIGHT WEEKS TO OPTIMUM HEALTH
A Proven Program for Taking Full Advantage
of Your Body's Natural Healing Power

EATING WELL FOR OPTIMUM HEALTH
The Essential Guide to Food, Diet, and Nutrition

THE HEALTHY KITCHEN
Recipes for a Better Body, Life, and Spirit
(*with Rosie Daley*)

HEALTHY AGING
A Lifelong Guide to Your Physical
and Spiritual Well-Being

The Marriage
of the
Sun and Moon

Dispatches from the
Frontiers of Consciousness

Andrew Weil, M.D.

Houghton Mifflin Company
Boston · New York

Visit our Web site: www.houghtonmifflinbooks.com.

Library of Congress Cataloging-in-Publication Data
Weil, Andrew.
The marriage of the sun and moon.
Bibliography: p.
Includes index.
ISBN 0-395-91154-0 (pbk.)
ISBN 0-618-47905-8 (pbk.)
1. Mind and body. 2. Consciousness. 3. Drugs —
Psychological aspects. I. Title.
BF161.W35 154.4 80-16603

Printed in the United States of America

QUM 10 9 8 7 6 5 4 3 2 1

The following chapters in this book previously appeared in various publications: "Throwing
Up in Mexico," in *High Times;* "Coffee Break," in *Journal of Psychedelic Drugs;* "When It's Mango
Time Down South," in *Journal of Altered States of Consciousness* and *High Times;* "Eating Chilies,"
in *Journal of Psychedelic Drugs* and *Harper's Weekly;* "A Good Fit," in *Journal of Psychedelic Drugs;*
"Mushrooms I," in *Journal of Altered States of Consciousness;* "Mushrooms II" and "Mushrooms
III" in *Journal of Psychedelic Drugs* and *Journal of Altered States of Consciousness;* "In the Land of
Yagé," in *Journal of Altered States of Consciousness* and *High Times;* "Is Heroin as Dangerous as
White Sugar?" in *Journal of Psychedelic Drugs, High Times,* and *The Diner's Club Way* (published
in Colombia); "The Green and the White," in *Journal of Psychedelic Drugs* and *Journal of Altered
States of Consciousness,* and in *The Coca Leaf and Cocaine Papers,* edited by George Andrews and
David Solomon (Harcourt Brace Jovanovich); "Some Notes on Datura," in *Journal of Psychedelic
Drugs;* "The Love Drug," in *Journal of Psychedelic Drugs;* "Now You See It, Now You Don't: The
Magic of Uri Geller," in *Psychology Today;* "When the Sun Dies," in *Harper's;* "The Marriage of the
Sun and Moon," in *Alternate States of Consciousness,* edited by Norman E. Zinberg, copyright ©
1977 by the Free Press, a Division of Macmillan Publishing Co., Inc.

And God made two great lights: the greater light to rule the day and the lesser light to rule the night . . .

—Genesis 1:16

Consider this: By an extraordinary coincidence, the sun and moon appear to us to be the same size in the sky. The sun's vast distance from us exactly compensates for its much greater diameter, so that it appears no bigger than the moon. If this relationship did not hold, total eclipses of the sun would not occur. Human consciousness has developed on the one planet where the lights that rule the day and night are equal.

Acknowledgments

The Institute of Current World Affairs made my travels possible and provided a haven in the middle of New York City. I thank the members and staff of that foundation, especially Dick Nolte, Jane Hartwig, Maria De-Benigno, and Theano Nikitas. For other assistance in getting around, I thank the editors of *High Times* and Tony Jones of *Harper's*.

For good company during some of my wanderings, I am grateful to Winnie Rosen, Woody Wickham, Peggy Sankot, and Chris Hall. People who took me in and made me welcome in distant places included Katha Sheehan and Margarita Dalton of El Vergel, Oaxaca, Mexico; Jorge Fuerbringer of Mocoa, Colombia; Leonard Crow Dog and family at Crow Dog's Paradise, Rosebud Reservation, South Dakota; Dean Ornish, Don Lohr, Dick Felger, Norman and Dorothy Zinberg, Tim and Jane Gold, Jeff Steingarten and Caron Smith, Jonathan Meader, the late Spencer Smith, the late Jack Wintz, David and Alice Smith, and the people of Camutí, Vaupés Territory, Colombia.

The following persons provided information that went into this book: Dick Schultes and the staff of the Harvard Botanical Museum; R. Gordon Wasson, Jesús M. Idrobo, Freda Morris, Eden Lipson, Tim Plowman, Jerry Beaver, Jonathan Ott, Daniel Stuntz, Georgy-M. Ola'h, Gastón Guzmán, Gary Nabhan, Greg McNamee, Richard Stone, Richard Leavitt, Sally Allen, Bob Harris, Jay Pasachoff, Jeremy Bigwood, Barry Zack, Richard Schweid, Steve Shouse, G. K. Sharma, Thomas E. Mails, James Randi, Diego León Giraldo, Silvia Patiño, Enrique Hernández; the staff of the Empresa Nacional de la Coca in Lima, Peru; and Msgr. Belarmino Correa Yepes of Mitú, Colombia.

I must thank Dan and Jenny for not worrying too much about me. And, finally, I thank Mahina for constant love, support, and help.

Preface to the New Edition

In reading over the chapters that make up this book, I thought it might be interesting to provide readers with updates on the subjects I wrote about three decades ago.

Conscious control of involuntary functions of the body ("Throwing Up in Mexico") remains mysterious, but there is growing recognition that imbalances of the autonomic nervous system underlie many common disease conditions, especially of the gastrointestinal tract. Irritable bowel syndrome (IBS) was not a defined clinical entity in the early 1970s; today it is a common diagnosis, as is GERD (gastro-esophageal reflux disorder). Allopathic medicine does not manage these problems well, because it ignores the mind-body interactions that are usually the cause of autonomic nervous system malfunction. Integrative approaches are much more successful. (See www.drweil.com for detailed recommendations.)

When I wrote "Coffee Break" way back when, espresso was something one tasted in Italy, and Seattle was not the latte capital of North America. If stronger and better forms of coffee are now bestsellers here, the big scientific news about stimulant beverages concerns tea. Tea turns out to have health benefits that coffee does not. It contains powerful antioxidants, notably EGCG (epigallo-catechin gallate), that reduce risks of heart disease, cancer, and other chronic illnesses. All teas contain these compounds, but green and white teas, being less processed than black tea, have more of them. Tea consumption is increasing in North America, and much better quality leaves are now available – in Asian grocery stores, teashops, and on the Internet. (Check out www.tea-health.co.uk for more information.)

I am happy to report that supplies of mangoes have improved also. It is now possible to get good, ripe mangoes here, at least some of the time, and decent mango sorbet is sold in most supermarkets. This is nothing compared to the phenomenal increase in chile consumption by Americans. A few years ago, sales of hot sauce surpassed sales of ketchup, something I would never have imagined, and the numbers and variety of chile products available are nothing short of astounding. (See www.mohotta.com, for example.) Spicy ethnic food has also become wildly popular, especially with the inroads made by the cuisines of Thailand, Vietnam, Hunan (China), and Korea. Moreover, medical science has found that capsaicin is a remarkable and long-acting local anesthetic. It is a focus of research in neurophysiology and a new remedy for such painful conditions as post-herpetic neuralgia, a complication of shingles.

I do not have much more to say about laughter than what I originally wrote in "A Good Fit," except to mention the appearance in India of a "laughter guru," Dr. Medan Kataria, a physician from Mumbai. Dr. Kataria launched his "laughter yoga" movement in 1995. There are now more than four hundred laughter clubs on the Indian subcontinent, and Dr. Kataria's disciples have founded similar clubs throughout the world. (See www.laughteryoga.org.) Participants meet regularly for group laughing sessions in order to promote physical and mental health. I am delighted to see an idea I had back in the 1970s come to such delightful fruition.

Mushrooms — magic and otherwise — have been much in the news. New species of *Psilocybe* continue to be discovered in North America; I am honored to have one named for me. *Psilocybe weilii* was first reported from Atlanta, Georgia, and is now abundant there. In 2002 researchers at the University of Arizona got permission to give psilocybin to human subjects as a novel treatment for obsessive-compulsive disorder (OCD). The study was prompted by reports of relief of OCD in patients who had used magic mushrooms. More important is the growing body of evidence for medicinal effects of mushrooms, particularly of species from China, Korea, and Japan that have long been valued as longevity tonics and enhancers of immunity. I now frequently recommend extracts of these mushrooms to patients with cancer, AIDS, and other chronic infectious illnesses. (Look up information on medicinal mushrooms at www.fungi.com and www.drweil.com.) I am also pleased to note that we share more DNA sequences with mushrooms than with plants and are thus more closely related to them.

I cannot believe that we are still stuck in the same pointless war against marijuana that we were when I wrote this book. This plant has clearly established itself as the most widely used illegal drug in our society, but efforts to decriminalize its possession and use continue to polarize us. Current battles rage over medical marijuana, with the federal government pitted against a growing number of states that have authorized its use for patients with cancer, AIDS, multiple sclerosis, and other conditions. It appears that those invested in the concept of marijuana as an evil weed cannot bear the thought that it has any redeeming qualities.

As for *yagé* – once an obscure and exotic psychedelic from the Amazon – it is now easily available in North America and highly regarded as a plant "ally" for people seeking spiritual growth, psychological benefit, and medical cure. Under its Peruvian name, *ayahuasca,* it is offered up in both secular and religious ceremonies here. The latter are offshoots of two new religions from Brazil, the Uniao do Vegetal, or UDV (see www.csp .org/nicholas-/A18.html), and Santo Daime (www.santodaime.org), which use ayahuasca as a sacrament. Both groups have survived numerous legal challenges in Brazil and are flourishing. The former are conducted by shamans, both traditional ones – Native Americans who travel here from Ecuador and Peru – and homegrown ones who have learned how to use the psychedelic potion. (For more information, go to www.thebrazilian.sound.com/ayahuasc.htm.)

And then there is sugar, probably more despised than ever with the rise in popularity of low-carbohydrate diets (Atkins, The Zone, Sugar Busters, etc.). Although mainstream medicine continues to reject the dietary philosophy behind these fads, it is slowly embracing a new and useful concept, the glycemic index, or GI. This is a rating of carbohydrate foods by how quickly they digest and raise levels of blood sugar (glucose). Regular consumption of high-GI foods stresses the pancreas and in many people leads to insulin resistance, obesity, and a tendency to develop type 2 dia-

betes. High-GI carbohydrates are prominent in the fast foods and
snacks that Americans love, and they appear to be a major factor
in the obesity epidemic here. It is worth noting, however, that table
sugar (sucrose) is intermediate on the GI because it consists of
a molecule of glucose linked to one of fructose (fruit sugar).
Although glucose is at the top of the GI scale, fructose is quite low
on it; it does not digest quickly or easily. (See www.glycemicindex
.com.)

I wish I had better news about coca and cocaine, but I am sorry
to report that ignorance of the differences between the plant and
its isolated alkaloid continues to drive our thinking and policies.
Cocaine use became epidemic in America among the affluent and
educated in the late 1970s and early 1980s, and the smoking of
crack cocaine appeared in the underclasses with devastating effects. Public alarm led directly to the War on Drugs that has continued for the past twenty years with little, predictably, to show for
all the effort. Cocaine use has all but disappeared from middle-
and upper-class America, but there is no evidence that use of illegal stimulants has decreased in the population. And the United
States continues to push for eradication of coca, with horrendous
consequences to the producing countries of South America, especially Colombia, Peru, and Bolivia. In short, I see no progress.

I have nothing to add to "Some Notes on *Datura*" except to note
that I have become an avid grower of Brugmansias, which turn
out to be quite easy to cultivate, are rewarding beyond measure in
their beauty, and are now plentifully available in a remarkable
range of hybrids. The forms and colors of the abundant flowers
are arresting. (See www.brugmansias.org.)

The "love drug," MDA, has vanished, but its shorter-acting derivative, MDMA, or ecstasy, has become the most popular recreational drug in the world. It is the fuel of the rave, that phenomenon of the late twentieth century that attracts the youth of
countries as diverse as China, Israel, and those of the United King-
dom, as well as the United States. Despite dire warnings from drug
warriors about neurotoxicity, it remains to be shown that occasional use of MDMA is harmful, and many psychotherapists are
enthusiastic about its potential to move people through emotional
quagmires. It appears to be a useful treatment for post-traumatic

stress disorder, for example. (See www.maps.org/research/mdma/;
www.mdma.net; and www.erowid.org/chemicals/mdma/mdma
.shtml.)

I don't hear much about iridology these days. It seems to have
dropped out of favor, even among practitioners of alternative
medicine, which is just as well. Of course, the popularity of alternative medicine has never been higher, and much of my work in
the past twenty-five years has been directed toward integrating
the ideas and practices of conventional and alternative systems of
treatment. (See www.integrativemedicine.arizona.edu.)

A few years ago I visited Uri Geller at his home on the Thames
west of London. He had just written a book about healing, containing sensible advice about a healthy lifestyle. Although he is not
much on the performance circuit these days, he continues to consult with people around the world, including scientists, and there
is a great deal of scientific interest in documenting the effects
of "subtle" energies on physical systems (www.issseem.org). The
National Institutes of Health has even funded a major research
center at the University of Arizona to investigate the human "bio-
field." (See www.biofield.arizona.edu.)

I have seen the sun die in a number of places around the world,
including Peru, Aruba, and Romania. I opted not to try for the
most recent event in Antarctica, but I see some tempting solar
eclipses coming up between 2005 and 2010. I still find them awe-
some. I have also been in many more sweat lodges. Remarkably
the Sioux (or Lakota) religion has had a great revival at the end of
the twentieth century, and many people around the world have
had a chance to experience the ritual of the sweat lodge.

Needless to say, I have not lost my interest in consciousness and
the unification of the mind. And I am still and always will be a
seeker.

Andrew Weil

Vail, Arizona
January 2004

Contents

	Acknowledgments	*vii*
	Preface to the New Edition	*ix*
	Preface to the 1998 Edition	*xv*
1.	Departure	1
2.	Throwing Up in Mexico	8
3.	Coffee Break	15
4.	When It's Mango Time Down South	23
5.	Eating Chilies	28
6.	A Good Fit	37
7.	Mushrooms I	43
8.	Mushrooms II	58
9.	Mushrooms III	73
10.	Marijuana Reconsidered	87
11.	In the Land of Yagé	99
12.	Is Heroin as Dangerous as White Sugar?	132
13.	The Green and the White: Coca and Cocaine	139
14.	Some Notes on *Datura*	166
15.	The Love Drug	177
16.	Reading the Windows of the Soul	181
17.	Now You See It, Now You Don't: The Magic of Uri Geller	191
18.	When the Sun Dies	222
19.	The Marriage of the Sun and Moon	241
	Glossary	*263*
	Suggested Reading	*273*
	Index	*277*

Preface to the 1998 Edition

Twenty-five years have passed since the events that are reported in these pages took place. My life today is very different from what it was when I was wandering the hemisphere in El Rojo, and I often look back on that time with nostalgia, as a relatively carefree period when life was simpler. All of my possessions were in my Land Rover; I was mostly my own boss; and I was out to discover new frontiers.

Today, I run a large and growing organization, have many responsibilities as a faculty member of a medical school, and find it hard to get a day off to go hiking, much less to make a major trip. I am developing new models of medical education and trying to create a new field, Integrative Medicine, that combines the best ideas and practices of conventional and alternative medicine while emphasizing the body's own innate power to heal itself. I also try to give people of all ages and all levels of education the information they need to keep themselves healthy.

I am frequently asked, "When did you convert to this way of thinking?" The assumption is that a physician could not come to believe in natural medicine except by way of a conversion experience such as a personal health crisis. I never had such a crisis. The fact is that I always thought this way, as far back as I can remember. My interest in plants began in early childhood, as did my interest in the mind and consciousness. Before I even entered medical school, I had started to look at other forms of healing.

But if there was any sort of watershed in my career it was somewhere in the course of the travels described in this book. Living with traditional peoples, learning about their plants, and experiencing how different ways of perceiving reality change reality all formed the foundation that underlies my present mission to re-store the connection between medicine and nature and empower patients and others to take greater charge of their destinies.

It is a pleasure to introduce this book to a new generation of readers.

Tucson, Arizona
January 1998

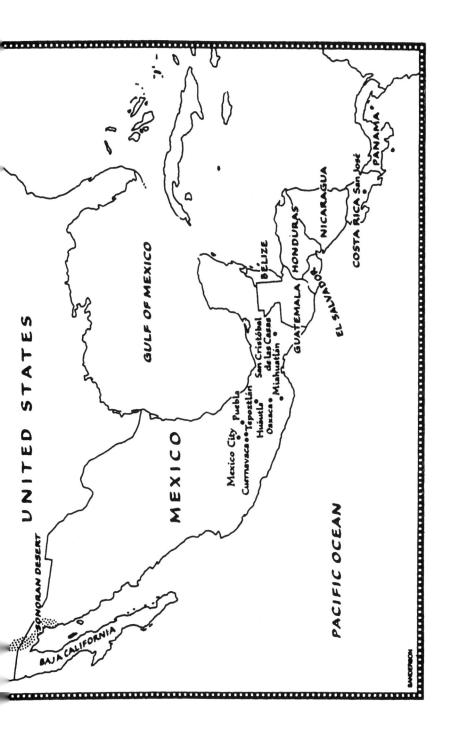

UNITED STATES

SONORAN DESERT

BAJA CALIFORNIA

MEXICO

GULF OF MEXICO

Mexico City Puebla
Cuernavaca Tepoztlán
Huautla
Oaxaca Miahuatlán

San Cristóbal
de las Casas

BELIZE

GUATEMALA

EL SALVADOR

HONDURAS

NICARAGUA

COSTA RICA San José

PANAMA

PACIFIC OCEAN

SANDERSON

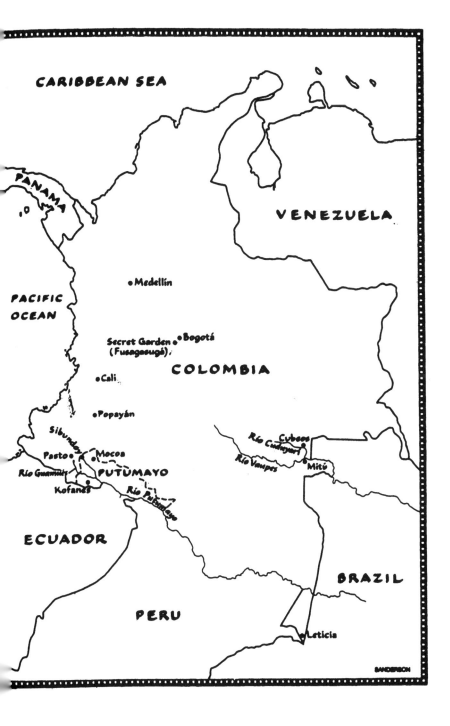

CARIBBEAN SEA

PANAMA

VENEZUELA

PACIFIC
OCEAN

• Medellín

Secret Garden • • Bogotá
(Fusagasugá)

COLOMBIA

• Cali

• Popayán

Sibundoy

Pasto • • Mocoa

Río Guamuéz

Kofanes

PUTUMAYO

Río Putumayo

Río Cuduyari   • Cubeos

Río Vaupes   • Mitú

ECUADOR

PERU

BRAZIL

• Leticia

SANDERSON

The Marriage of the Sun and Moon

1

DEPARTURE

On a violently stormy night in September 1971 I left my house near Sterling, Virginia, to drive to New Jersey on the first leg of a journey that would take four years and cover many thousands of miles. I rode north through blinding rain in a 1969 red Land Rover I had just acquired. It would soon be known to me as El Rojo and was to be a faithful companion through the mountains, deserts, and jungles of North and South America.

Sometimes we cross divides in our lives that are visible only in retrospect, being unaware at the time that an action taken or a parting is to mark the end of one phase and the opening of another. But that night in the blackness of northern Virginia was planned and anticipated as an important transition. I had put my affairs in order, packed up or given away most of my possessions, reduced my material needs to what I could fit in the back of El Rojo, and had prepared my body and mind for a long trip into the unknown.

For the previous year I had lived by myself in rural Loudoun County, enjoying the country, learning to be quiet, and working on the manuscript of a book. I finished the book in August and delivered it to the publisher just before leaving. It would appear a year later as *The Natural Mind: A New Way of Looking at Drugs and the Higher Consciousness*. In it I set out a theory of drugs and the mind based on several years of research, experience, and observation. Much of the book was speculative, the product of periods of reflection in the Virginia woods and the ordering of a great deal of information I had compiled during my medical training and my work as a researcher. On finishing the book, I was eager to go out in the world again and test my theories, to see more, have new experiences, and refine my ideas.

I was enabled to do that by a remarkable foundation in New York City called the Institute of Current World Affairs, which awarded me a fellowship to travel about and collect information on altered states of consciousness, drug use in other cultures, and other matters to do with the complementarity of mind and body. The night that I drove to New Jersey was the start of my new life as a fellow of that institute.

During the years that I held this position, the institute provided me with full financial support. In return I had two obligations. The first was to write a brief report twice a year summarizing my activities. The second was to write, on the average of one a month, newsletters on topics of my investigations. These were to be addressed to the executive director of the institute, Mr. Richard H. Nolte, for reproduction and private circulation to a list of my friends and a list of "certain persons in government, education, business, and the professions" who were interested in me or in the area about which I would be writing.

In the course of my fellowship, I wrote thirty-nine of these newsletters. They were mailed to New York from a variety of stopping points and covered a broad range of subjects. Some of them have since appeared in scientific journals and popular magazines. These newsletters, edited and revised, are published here for the first time in book form.

My fellowship was a bit unusual. Most institute fellows go to a particular region of the world, stay there for several years, and write about it. I moved about constantly and investigated a general theme rather than a geographical area. That the subject matter of my investigations qualified as a "current world affair" reflected the growing interest in consciousness at all levels of society at the beginning of the 1970s, as well as the willingness of Dick Nolte to be innovative and unconventional.

My favorite method of research is participant observation.

I like to experience people and activities, record my impressions, and then analyze them at leisure. The fellowship provided an excellent opportunity for that kind of work, and the newsletters a perfect format for recording it.

There were several questions I hoped to look at in my travels, all of them raised by theories in *The Natural Mind*. In the first place, I wanted to observe the relationships traditional peoples form with psychoactive plants. Second, I wanted to think about ways of getting high and changing consciousness without drugs. Third, I wanted to sharpen my conceptions of mind-body interactions and their implications for health and medicine.

The first of these topics reflects my long-standing interests in curious plants, New World Indians, herbal medicine, and psychoactive drugs. I needed to see certain plants firsthand and learn their uses from people who had lived with them for generations. One reason for doing so was to test my theory that some Indians have solved the problem of drug abuse by allowing ritualized use of natural drugs in positive ways under careful social controls. Accordingly, many of the pieces in this book are descriptions of plants that affect the mind and of people who use them to change their awareness of themselves and the world.

But the concerns of this book are broader than drugs, and I hope readers will notice that I am writing about drugs mainly as models of interactions between human consciousness and natural forces. Long ago, I came to understand that people's expectations of drugs often explain their responses to them better than books of pharmacology; psychologists call this kind of expectation "set." Social and cultural setting also modify pharmacology. Over and over in my research and writing, I have stressed the importance of set and setting. Furthermore, drugs are typical of many elements in nature that are both powerful and ambivalent. They can either harm us or help us. The choice seems to be ours: Drugs become useful or dangerous depending on how we view them and how we use them.

The chapters describing drug plants are really about set

and setting, conceptual models, and the power of mind to modify physical reality. For example, these same ideas apply to phenomena like fire walking and healing, which are also discussed here. How is it possible for people to handle fire and not get burned? Why do unorthodox medical treatments based on absurd theories sometimes cure patients of real diseases, while rational, scientific treatments sometimes fail? Belief is the key to these mysteries: not intellectual conviction but gut-level belief that links up with the physical nervous system and, through it, influences all the functions of the body.

The catch in this scheme is that the kind of belief that matters is often unconscious and may be at variance with conscious belief. People may tell you they expect thus and so of a drug or a medical treatment, but they may expect something quite different at the level of mind that connects to the nervous system and be unaware of it. This problem has led me to consider the nature of the unconscious mind and its relationship to the ordinary mind.

A major theme of *The Natural Mind* was that people take drugs to produce desired altered states of consciousness, to get high. But the highs of drug experience seem essentially the same as highs obtained through music, dancing, sex, athletics, meditation, hypnosis, religious ecstasy, and many other activities. I concluded that highs are innate capacities of the nervous system and that drugs merely trigger them by making us feel physically different, thereby giving us opportunities to be high. For this reason, drugs do not work unless set and setting encourage us to interpret their direct physical effects in ways that allow us to be high. Also, I suggested that the neurological basis of high states is some sort of interchange between the conscious and unconscious minds, between higher and lower parts of the brain.

The statement that highs can be had without drugs (and may be better that way because they are uncontaminated by irrelevant effects on the body) brought me much criticism from committed users and researchers of drugs. Some of these people insisted that drug highs were special in some way, either more intense or more interesting than nondrug highs.

I heard this objection so often that I began to wonder if I were mistaken. Had I myself ever had as intense an experience without a drug as with LSD, for example? Certainly my clumsy skill at meditation had not brought me anything approaching an LSD trip. Yet two experiences seemed to me to qualify: learning the ritual of the Indian sweat lodge from a Sioux medicine man in South Dakota and seeing a total eclipse of the sun in southern Mexico. So powerful were these highs that I was eager to repeat them. At the start of my travels with El Rojo, I went back to South Dakota for more of the sweat lodge, and in 1973 I caught another solar eclipse in Africa.

The eclipses suggested to me a model of consciousness I found very useful. I took the sun and moon as symbols of the two spheres of the mind, and a total eclipse as the symbol of a union that produces transcendent states. This theme is developed in "The Marriage of the Sun and Moon," the last chapter, which also describes the sweat lodge. All of the chapters converge toward the idea of unifying consciousness.

*

I knew that Latin America would be a rich source of information. Therefore, I went to Mexico to learn Spanish. Once in Mexico, at the beginning of November, I quickly abandoned my plan to take formal language classes in Cuernavaca and settled, instead, in the nearby village of Tepoztlán. There I became one of the first students in a new, experimental school called the Colegio de Tepoztlán, under the direction of Marco Polansky, an offbeat teacher and unforgettable character. Marco, an Italian Jew who had lived in Israel and Sweden, now was based in Tepoztlán with an American wife and daughter, two Italian daughters by a previous marriage, and an adopted Mexican son. His household was a polyglot's delight.

Marco's philosophy of learning languages was out of the ordinary but struck me as correct. He said we all had the capacity to learn languages, since we did it as infants, that it had nothing to do with intellect but rather was an operation of the unconscious mind. The only abilities it depended upon were accurate listening and accurate imitating. Therefore, the way to learn a new language is to want to learn it badly and to immerse yourself in it, letting as much of it flow into the unconscious mind as possible; whether you understand it or not is irrelevant. Forget about grammar books and formal instruction, Marco said. Just listen and imitate.

"Classes" at the Colegio de Tepoztlán were bizarre. Sometimes Marco would have us fall into trance states to the accompaniment of recorded chamber music while he intoned vocabulary words from a Spanish comic book. When pressed for more-structured help, he would decline, saying there was no way to teach another person a language. He did arrange for us to be apprenticed to local people to force us to talk. I was placed in the care of the village carpenter, who was also the mail carrier, and spent many pleasant afternoons with him in an outdoor shop, helping to make furniture.

I must say that the Polansky method worked like a charm. In three months I was speaking passable Spanish, and three months after that (I was in Colombia by then) I was speaking good Spanish. The only other language I ever learned as well was German, and that took four years of painful work in high school. I would never again attempt to learn a language by studying it, and I have no doubt that I can learn any language now just by really wanting to and placing myself in the right part of the world. I am grateful to Marco for teaching me that lesson.

Tepoztlán was a fine place to live. It had a colorful Indian market, delightfully eccentric gringos, and spectacular mountains: the Sierra Tepozteco, named for the Aztec god of *pulque* and intoxication. (Pulque is the traditional fermented drink made from the sap of the blue maguey.) A rugged climb from the village led to a pyramid used for worship of the god. My coming to Tepozteco's sacred spot to begin my fellowship seemed curiously appropriate.

At the beginning of February 1972 with the coming of the

period of "crazy weather" (*febrero loco* is the Mexican term), on an afternoon of fierce winds, green thunderheads, and salmon and purple light on the mountains of Tepozteco, I readied El Rojo for the next move. At the first light of dawn, I drove off to the Mazatec region of northeast Oaxaca to encounter the famed magic mushrooms and then continue south to Central America and Colombia.

2

THROWING UP IN MEXICO

VOMITING IS NOT a subject for polite discussion, at least not around the dinner table. Nevertheless, I consider it an important subject because it has much to teach us about the relationships between mind and body and the natural mechanisms available to us for altering internal processes. Also, it provides an example of how physical realities can be changed by adopting different mental conceptions of them. Finally, it offers some practical clues about possibilities of coordinating conscious and unconscious mental energies.

A good place to begin is with the very emotional attitudes that stand in the way of our talking about vomiting in polite company. Vomiting is an ultimately antisocial act in societies desirous of relegating natural functions to the obscurity of the lavatory, away from public view. Moreover, these attitudes seem to be justified by experience; most of us have vomited only in association with illness and do not think of it as something we could feel good about, let alone practice openly.

That such feelings are not universal may come as a surprise to many persons. But, for example, instructional materials on yoga urge students to learn to vomit voluntarily, to practice it regularly, and to perform it as a morning ritual (called *jala dhauti*), much as many people gargle. American Indians who eat hallucinogenic plants that cause nausea often vomit effortlessly and unself-consciously. Vomiting is even a central part of certain Indian rituals, such as the sahuaro wine festival of the Papagos, held near the summer solstice in the Sonoran Desert along the Mexico-United States border. The Papagos force themselves to drink as much as possible of a fresh wine made from the sweet, red fruit of giant cactuses. The vomiting and urinating that follow are supposed to help bring on the summer rains and thereby ensure survival through the hottest season.

In my medical training I was taught nothing about vomiting except as a symptom of disease, but I do not regret having learned that information. For it is my understanding of the nervous mechanisms underlying the process that makes me so willing to pay attention to what yogis say are the right uses of those mechanisms. Vomiting is a reflex action. That is, it is initiated by nervous impulses from the periphery of the body (usually the stomach), which, traveling to a center in the brain, produce an outgoing nervous impulse that causes the regurgitation of stomach contents. Now, the vomiting center is in an anatomically discrete part of the brain called the medulla oblongata, the connecting link between the lowest portion of the brainstem and the uppermost portion of the spinal cord. Because it also contains centers regulating heartbeat and respiration, the medulla may be considered the most vital unit of the entire nervous system whose disruption means cessation of the life of the body. Occasionally, vomiting arises directly from irritation of the medulla itself in the absence of impulses from the stomach: so-called "central vomiting," which may be a symptom of serious trouble in the brain. Because the medulla is that part of the brain farthest from the cortex and closest to the spinal cord, and because its centers control the basic rhythms of life, which will continue even in deep coma, neurologists think of it as a keystone of the involuntary nervous system.

The nerve fibers that issue from the vomiting center in the medulla to the alimentary tract form part of the vagus nerve, a huge conduit that leaves the cranium to innervate many structures in the throat, chest, and abdomen. The vagus is a principal component of the parasympathetic nervous system — that portion of the autonomic system whose influence is to slow down certain internal functions and conserve energy. For example, when vagal fibers to the heart are stimulated, heartbeat slows down. During the act of vomiting, massive vagal discharges occur, producing a number of physiological changes in addition to emptying of the stomach. Is it possible that learning to vomit willfully opens this important channel of unconscious activity to conscious influence? Might it not also extend cortical influence to the very center of the unconscious part of the brain, the medulla?

I think the answer to both questions is yes. These neurological considerations make me inclined to listen carefully to Easterners who say that learning to vomit at will is a beneficial exercise. Eastern systems of mind development like yoga are based in subjective experience of internal states, not in neurology, and often yogic conceptions of the nervous system are fanciful. By contrast, we in the West know much about neurological mechanisms but often very little about their correlations with experience. What is the significance of the *experience* of the vomiting reflex and what is its purpose?

I have seen vomiting function to change conscious experience dramatically in three ways:

It can be a means of ridding the body of unwanted materials. Vomiting often brings instant relief and a sense of well-being to someone who has ingested substances that the body does not want to accept, such as toxins. It is worth recalling that the inside of the stomach is actually outside the body because it is continuous with the exterior, and that substances have not entered the body until they cross the walls of the stomach or the intestines and pass into the bloodstream. Vomiting merely shunts materials that are already outside the body back to a point where absorption into the body cannot occur. Anyone who has experienced this knows how rapid can be the transition from sickness to health.

Vomiting can be a way of discharging unwanted sensations from the body. Occasionally, in the absence of ingestion of toxins, vomiting can serve as a powerful cure of such conditions as motion sickness and headache, particularly if undigested food remains in the stomach. Many people experience relief of seasickness as soon as they can throw up. Probably, fewer have learned how to get rid of headache by the same means. A young Indian man I met in Tepoztlán described this method to me: If a headache is so severe as to be incapacitating, it can be eliminated in three steps. First, while lying down with the eyes closed, create in the mind's eye a visual image of the pain, preferably with discrete form, color, and location. Second, again using the visual imagination, transfer the image to the stomach. Third, stand up and expel the pain by vomiting. Of course, this technique assumes some mastery of the art of vomiting.

It can also be used as a means of ejecting unwanted emotions from the mind. That vomiting may have mental or spiritual applications may seem strange. Quite commonly, however, people who take psychedelic intoxicants experience nausea and anxiety at the onset of drug effects. The sooner they can vomit, the sooner they can get into a high state of consciousness. Many natural hallucinogens — peyote is a good example — are supposed to trigger nausea by their direct pharmacological actions. Yet Indians who eat peyote regularly may not become nauseated. Other drugs are not known to be nauseating by virtue of their pharmacology, yet some people who try them experience severe nausea that is relieved by vomiting. Having watched many people take many drugs, I feel that nausea at the onset of the effect of hallucinogens is a physical analogue of mental resistance to "letting go" — of extreme anxiety about detaching oneself from the ordinary consciousness of the ego in order to experience reality in another way. By concentrating this resistance and anxiety in the form of physical sensations in the stomach and then expelling them by vomiting, a person can cure himself of these unwanted emotions.

How difficult is it to learn to use this natural mechanism, and what are the obstacles to mastering it? Much of the difficulty is mental rather than physical. Until one gets over the idea that vomiting is unnatural, unpleasant, and wrong, one cannot begin to work the autonomic controls that nature has given us. People I have met who have mastered the technique say that when isolated from these negative interpretations, the physical act of vomiting becomes a pleasant, natural sensation that promotes a feeling of health. Many methods are available for learning the process, from drinking quantities of salt water to inducing retching with a finger in the throat, but the goal is to be able to vomit quietly, smoothly, and with as few external aids as possible. Women seem to have less difficulty than men, possibly because they are more willing to abandon themselves to internal sensations.

Over the past years in the course of my own work at yoga, I have practiced vomiting with sporadic success and intend to keep going. I found it difficult at the outset but easier with practice. When attempting to vomit, I have found it useful to remind myself that I am not trying to remove material from inside my body, merely trying to move material already outside. I have also found proper mental imagery to be helpful. Part of the secret of getting hold of the medullary vomiting center seems to be imagining that mechanism at work — that is, holding in mind an image of a focus at the base of the brain that is connected to the stomach in just the right way to make vomiting possible.

Once you can initiate the reflex, the problem is to control it. The involuntary muscle spasms are violent and painful at first until you learn to balance them by using your voluntary muscles. It is easiest to vomit when you genuinely want to remove something from your stomach; ice cream is the best food to practice with. If you vomit within thirty minutes of eating, food tastes the same on the way up as on the way down. There is no sourness or other unpleasant flavor.

From the successes I have had, I can testify that the result is indeed a feeling of well-being. One side effect, for example, is a profound stimulation of respiration, possibly a consequence of exercising the medulla. Also, vomiting is usually accompanied by lacrimation, a further spillover of autonomic activity, and the sensation of tears freely pouring from the eyes is one I associate with invigoration and cleansing.

In Mexico I met a number of people interested in vomiting, including some who had very positive experiences of it. New World Indians and those who live close to them tend to be more accepting of bodily processes than most of us. At the same time, Indians, though they may be perfectly happy to vomit when they feel like it, may not have the knowledge of the nervous system to motivate them to acquire mastery of the process in a disciplined way. If we are to achieve harmony of mind and body, we must try to synthesize intellectual and experiential knowledge in a common framework. Like that of most physicians, my knowledge of the autonomic nervous system is mainly intellectual. I continue to practice vomiting as one means of complementing this knowledge with direct experience.

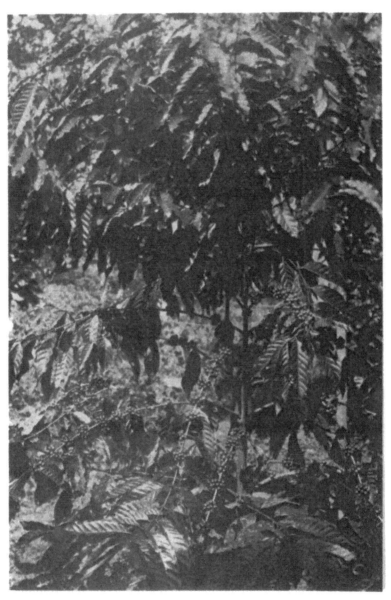

Coffee, *Coffea arabica*, is a small tree or shrub widely planted in the tropics. The fruits, called cherries, are red when ripe. Each contains two seeds, which become the coffee beans of commerce. (Courtesy Harvard Botanical Museum)

3

COFFEE BREAK

LATIN AMERICA is truly the land of caffeine. Three of the major caffeine-containing plants — coffee, cacao, and cola — are consumed there in vast quantities. Cola is native to Africa and is grown there and in the West Indies. It comes to Latin Americans in the form of the same brands of bottled cola beverages we are all familiar with in the United States. (Actually, these drinks have only small amounts of cola nut extract and are fortified with added caffeine from other sources.) Coffee is also an Old World native, believed to have originated in Abyssinia (now Ethiopia), but the American tropics are its adopted home. Countries like Guatemala are as much coffee republics as banana republics: A great human effort goes to growing, processing, exporting, and consuming the precious bean. Cacao — source of chocolate, cocoa, and cocoa butter — has been here all along. It was one of the New World's most treasured gifts to the Old.

Tea, whose home is China, is not much in evidence in Central America. But farther south, people drink two other caffeine beverages that are virtually unknown in the rest of the world. Maté or *yerba maté* is the national drink of Argentina; it is occasionally and erroneously sold in the United States as a variety of tea. Guaraná, obtained from the seeds of a jungle vine, is the base of the carbonated caffeine drink of Brazil, a beverage more popular than cola in that country.

But it is coffee that is always most visible. In the larger open markets of the Guatemalan highlands every other woman sells the gray-green unroasted beans, and the scent

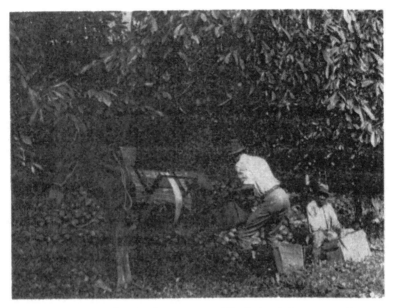

Harvesting cacao pods, *Theobroma cacao*. The fruit of these trees gives us chocolate, cocoa, and cocoa butter. (Courtesy Harvard Botanical Museum)

of finished coffee wafts out of many houses. It is *café* that has lent its name to a place where caffeine beverages of all sorts are sold, and café that has given its name to the stimulating alkaloid common to all of these important plants of commerce. Traveling through the coffee-producing regions of the Americas made me more conscious of the place of this substance in our world.

Except for cacao, which contains a high proportion of fat, none of these plants is nutritive; the drinks made from them supply nourishment only by virtue of added sugar or milk. It is worth thinking about how much energy has always gone into their cultivation, often in regions where nutrition is poor to begin with. The reason, of course, is that the products of these plants are drugs, not simple beverages or flavors, and the attention devoted to them is another example of the involvement with drugs that is so characteristic of human beings.

Caffeine itself is one member of a family of related compounds, the xanthines, that occur in various combinations in the different plants. All are stimulants and diuretics (that is, they promote the flow of urine). Theophylline, the principal xanthine in tea, is sometimes added to asthma medications because of its relaxant effect on bronchial smooth muscle. Caffeine is often included in proprietary compounds like "cold tablets" to offset the drowsiness induced by antihistamines or other components. But in general, these drugs have little specific clinical use today. We need not pay attention to the pharmacological distinctions within the family. For our purposes, caffeine can be considered the prototype of the xanthines. In fact, in their final forms of preparation, the beverages made from the different plants are roughly equivalent in caffeine content, so that a cup of coffee should be about as stimulating as a cup of tea or chocolate or a bottle of cola.

In practice, coffee seems to be much stronger and more toxic than its relatives. The explanation of this discrepancy may be that coffee contains other pharmacologically active substances that enhance the effect of caffeine. Unlike the other plants, coffee is rich in oil-soluble drugs, and these are little studied. We know much less than we should about how the effects of whole drug plants differ from those of their isolated "active principles," because pharmacologists for more than a century have taught that complex plants can be reduced to single compounds, and because contemporary pharmacologists and physicians have little interest in the plants, only in the pure chemicals derived from them. Coffee is one of many examples of drug plants that do somewhat different things to human beings from what their isolated chief constituents do. Possibly the oil-soluble fraction of coffee accounts for the differences, either through effects of its own or by synergism with caffeine.

Caffeine itself affects various parts of the body. The feeling of wakefulness and contentment that many people associate with it comes from stimulation of the central nervous system. In addition, caffeine activates voluntary muscle fibers, sometimes producing restlessness and jitteriness ("coffee nerves").* It may increase the flow of acid in the stomach, making it taboo for ulcer patients, and may stimulate intestinal mobility, sometimes causing diarrhea in sensitive persons who consume too much.

A problem in trying to describe these effects is that individuals vary greatly in their susceptibility to them, particularly to the central stimulation. Some people appear to be caffeine-resistant. For example, I have never been able to derive the least degree of alertness or wakefulness from coffee and can fall asleep after drinking any amount if I am tired to begin with. On the other hand, I know some people who cannot sleep at all during the night if they have so much as half a cup of coffee before retiring.

Pharmacologists have little to say about the reasons for these idiosyncratic variations — whether they represent physiological differences, for instance, in the body's ability to metabolize caffeine; or whether they are more results of differing expectations, possibly unconscious, of what the drug will do. In my own studies of drugs, I have seen again and again the power of expectation and environment to modify or overrule pharmacology. Therefore, I am inclined to think that with caffeine, as with all other drugs that affect mental function, individual variations in response might correlate with psychological differences as well as with physiological ones. The same is true, I think, of differences in patterns of use that form around psychoactive drugs: The same drug that one person can take or leave may become the object of extreme dependence for another.

In other words, the "addictive potential" of drugs is risky to discuss because the important variation is in the addictive potential of people, and for any drug — from heroin to coffee — there will exist a whole spectrum of human relationships with the drug, from casual and occasional use to frank addiction.

---

* This is different from the stimulation of amphetamines, which activate functional groups of muscles rather than individual muscle fibers. Both types of stimulants cause wakefulness, but amphetamines are more useful if one needs a chemical aid for functional motor acts like running or typing.

There is no doubt that true addictions do develop to the caffeine beverages. Indeed, I have seen many people have as much difficulty disengaging themselves from regular use of coffee as from tobacco, alcohol, or heroin. I also see many people who cannot begin to function in the morning until they have a sizable fix of coffee. Before they consume the drug, they cannot open their eyes fully, execute coordinated movements, or perform simple intellectual tasks. These symptoms are nothing other than classical pharmacological withdrawal: They appear when the organism is deprived of the drug during sleep and disappear as soon as the drug is reinstituted. Another common symptom of dependence on coffee is inability to move the bowels until the drug is taken.

People who are dependent on caffeine often get no positive effects from it. They are aware only of relief of negative symptoms — for example, the dissipation of mental cloudiness in the morning. In the same way, many opiate users come to enjoy relief of unpleasant symptoms of early withdrawal once they are regular users. Heavy users of caffeine beverages sometimes show a kind of restlessness and inability to maintain one position for more than a few seconds that may be a true pharmacological effect; it can be seen in animals given caffeine. Such restlessness is a prominent symptom of what I call the caffeine-nicotine syndrome, a common pattern of drug dependence in which heavy use of coffee and heavy use of cigarettes go together as expressions of neurotic anxiety. (This syndrome is almost universal at meetings of Alcoholics Anonymous but is never discussed.)

What is most curious about caffeine habits is that users are so often blind to the true nature of their dependence on the drug, a blindness that seems to result from a widely held social definition of caffeine preparations as beverages, not drugs. We have all grown up in a society that accepts completely and even encourages the regular use of caffeine. Since that society also defines drug use as bad, caffeine cannot be a drug. I have attended numerous conferences on the drug problem at which prodigious quantities of coffee were served and drunk without anyone noticing the incongruity.

Groups like the Mormons who shun coffee, tea, and cola as stimulants are distinctly in the minority.

This cultural blindness to the true nature of caffeine causes real problems. I have collected numerous cases of coffee toxicity that have gone undiagnosed just because many patients and doctors do not think of coffee as a possible influence on health. For example, I have gone over several reports of patients admitted to neurology wards of hospitals for evaluation of gross hand tremors, who were put through expensive and dangerous tests before anyone bothered to ask them about coffee intake. Some of these people were drinking thirty cups a day and more. Clearly, the coffee was the single cause of the tremors. I also see many women with chronic lower urinary tract complaints who have never been told by physicians that coffee might be a major contributor to their discomfort. Often these complaints subside as soon as coffee is discontinued, since women are particularly susceptible to the bladder-irritant effect of this substance.

I do not mean to imply that the United States has a monopoly on this strange way of perceiving (or, rather, not perceiving). Before leaving Mexico, I stayed for a while with an Indian family in the Sierra Mazateca of northeast Oaxaca, a center of coffee production. The coffee pot was started up early in the morning and was kept going until late at night. Throughout the day, all members of the family, from a two-year-old on up, drank the brew — strong, black, and full of sugar. Yet these people were outspoken in their criticism of what they called "drug users."

This process of social definition is a true form of magic, for it determines what we see and what we do not see. In objective terms, coffee is a stronger drug than marijuana, with a greater potential for toxicity. Both can be used to promote desired states of consciousness, and intelligent use of both is consistent with health and social productivity. Yet both can become objects of dependent behavior. Frankly, I have seen far more cases of full-blown coffee addiction than I have of marijuana addiction, and dependence on coffee has a much greater physiological component than dependence on marijuana. The most important difference between these two substances is that one enjoys full social support to the extent that its true identity as a drug is defined out of existence, while the other is thought of as something alien, dangerous, and menacing. When I stay at motels, attend drug conferences, or participate in morning rounds in hospitals, I am plied with free coffee. And when I worked briefly at the National Institute of Mental Health I was allowed to leave my desk periodically to have coffee — a legitimate excuse in the eyes of the federal government. If I smoke a joint publicly, in many places I can be thrown in jail as a threat to society — in Latin America just as in the United States.

When coffee was a relatively new discovery in the Middle East, early Muslim mystics used it ritually, reverently, and occasionally, to facilitate states of concentration and meditation. They did not become dependent on it and experienced no adverse effects on their health. Were coffee thought of as a drug in our society and treated with the respect that drugs demand, we might be able to use it that way, too, and our health as a nation would be better for the change. Similarly, marijuana, if used ritually, reverently, and occasionally, can be a temporary aid to the experience of other states of consciousness of potential benefit. It has been used this way by some Hindu mystics over the centuries. But as marijuana becomes a commonplace, as its use increases and people begin to think of it more as an herb for smoking than as a drug — in short, as it becomes as ordinary in the lives of Americans as coffee, it will gradually lose its power to transport its users to interesting realms of experience.

It is, perhaps, hard to imagine that coffee, too, was once a magic plant. Our ways of thinking about it have changed its nature. This is why pharmacology seems less interesting than psychology in considering drugs: The "effects" of psychoactive substances are relative to a particular time, place, and culture. They change as people's and societies' views of them change. If we can begin to understand the nature of this process, how objective reality can be changed by changing our conceptions of it, we might have a key for unlocking ourselves from many of the seemingly impossible social jams we are now in, including those with drugs.

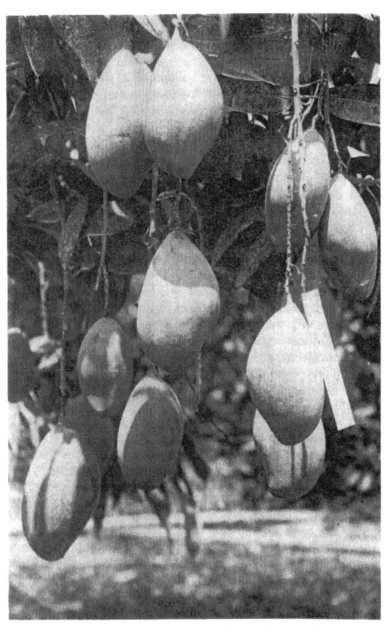

Mangoes, *Mangifera indica*, hang from branches in clusters. When ripe, they drop to the ground. (Courtesy Harvard Botanical Museum)

4

WHEN IT'S MANGO TIME
DOWN SOUTH

ARRIVING IN SAN JOSÉ, the capital of Costa Rica, I found
mangoes on sale on every downtown streetcorner. Big
mangoes. Ripe mangoes. Wonderful mangoes.

It will be hard for me to convey the joy of this discovery. I
have a passion for mangoes, and although I have traveled in
the tropics before, I have never managed to be in a mango-
growing region when the fruit was in season. In India, once,
I was too early; in South America, too late; in Mexico, too
early again. But this time I was not to be cheated. In southern Mexico in February I saw the first green mangoes on the
streets of San Cristóbal de las Casas. Unripe, the size of eggs,
and as hard as potatoes, they were sliced and eaten as
snacks with salt and chili. The taste is sour, bracingly sour,
yet with more than a hint of the distinctive flavor that is so
overwhelmingly delicious in the ripe fruit. In Guatemala
in early March I came across the first ripe ones. Small,
blotched, of uneven quality, they hardly deserved to be
called mangoes. But they were an unmistakable sign that I
was on the trail and getting warm.

Then San José! When I say there were mangoes on every
downtown streetcorner, I mean every downtown streetcorner. And there was not just one kind. I was able to buy four
varieties of mango in Costa Rica, each better than the last.
One was long, oval, yellow, and drippingly juicy. Another
was large, round, orange-red, with flesh the consistency of
ice cream. The flavor of each kind was different. Probably

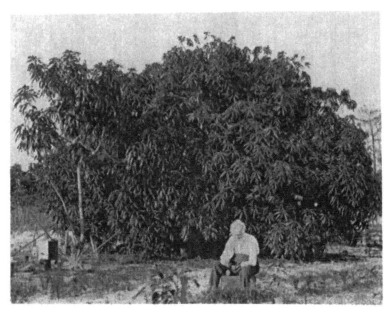

The dense shade of these beautiful mango trees is most welcome in the hot tropics where they grow. (Courtesy Harvard Botanical Museum)

that was just the beginning. There are hundreds of varieties of mango, and these were just the earliest.

My mango cravings go back to early childhood in Philadelphia when a fruitarian aunt let me taste one that had been sent to her from Florida. In those days mangoes hardly ever made it north. Now, they are shipped up quite regularly, so that even the rural farm market near my old home in northern Virginia had them in June. Of the mangoes that one can buy in the North, only a few are worth eating. Picked long before they are ripe, removed from the intense sun that they depend on, their maturation is aborted and they rarely ripen in the way nature intended. A mango that is not perfectly ripe is far from wonderful, for it contains a powerful concentration of acid and an oil that tastes like turpentine.* People

* The mango is a member of the cashew family, the Anacardiaceae, a plant group rich in toxins and irritant oils. Poison ivy belongs to this family. The skin of the mango contains an oil that produces in some people a contact dermatitis like that of poison ivy. Allergic individuals can still enjoy the fruit if they handle it with gloves and peel it carefully before eating.

who think they do not like mangoes may never have tasted one in the right stage for eating. To do that, one must really go to the tropics. For the mango is a tree of the torrid zone, and even in southern Florida it is not quite as happy as it should be.

The Asian tropics are the native home of the mango, and in Asia no country is more closely associated with the fruit than India, where the mango tree is regarded as sacred. The best mangoes in the world are said to come from Bombay. An Indian I met in Bombay told me that at the height of the season, people lie on the sidewalks with glazed looks of ecstasy as they let ripe mangoes drip into their mouths. In his *Autobiography of a Yogi*, the late Paramahansa Yogananda wrote that it is impossible for a Hindu to conceive of a heaven without mangoes. Recently I came across the following exchange between the great Hindu saint, Ramakrishna (1836–1886), and his chief disciple, Narendra:

NARENDRA: Is there no afterlife? What about punishment for our sins?

MASTER: Why not enjoy your mangoes? What need have you to calculate about the afterlife and what happens then and things like that? Eat your mangoes. You need mangoes.*

This reverence for mangoes is visible wherever they grow. One day in San José I bought a bag of them and went back to my hotel to eat them. The elevator boy asked me what I had bought. "Mangoes," I said. "Oh," he said, and we looked at each other and grinned. He knew. Mango vendors grin at you the same way. They know. They all know the capacity of this fruit to give extraordinary pleasure. A tugboat captain with whom I once shared some mangoes in Miami at the tail end of the season said as he slurped a juicy slice, "Next best thing to sex."

The flavor of the mango is neither subtle nor simple. It is complex and rich the way the music of India is complex. The fruit is so luscious that it commands one's whole attention. I

* Quoted in Philip Kapleau, *The Wheel of Death* (New York: Harper & Row, 1971), p. 57.

have seen people eat ordinary fruit — apples, oranges, bananas — casually, nibbling at them while reading, writing, carrying on conversations. I have never seen anyone eat a perfect mango and be able to do anything but concentrate on the pure pleasure of the experience. I indulged in that experience frequently during the week I spent in San José.

Now, although I could not do much thinking while I was actually experiencing these mango highs, I could not help noticing afterward how analogous they are to other sorts of highs. In fact, the image of Indians in Bombay stretched out with glazed expressions dripping mangoes into their mouths has always stuck with me because it sounds so much like an altered state of consciousness. The knowing grins of mango devotees, the comparison of the pleasure of eating the fruit to sexual pleasure, the sacred status of the tree in India, all point to an ability to transport people to a realm of experience out of the ordinary. The essence of that experience is concentration, in this case on an intensely pleasureful sensation in the mouth. When I indulge in serious mango eating, I become oblivious to what is around me, even to what is inside me, such as my thoughts. For a brief time there is nothing but the pleasure, and the pleasure is a high.

Or perhaps it would be better to say that the pleasure triggers a transcendent state, because it seems to me that it is the concentration that is the high, the pleasure being merely the stimulus for concentration. Anything that can bring about this focusing of attention can get us high, even if it is something normally perceived as painful. In fact, pain itself, if a person is set to perceive it differently (that is, to accept it, not to resist it), can bring about a state of intense concentration and a resultant experience of transcendence. The highs of altered states of consciousness such as those of trance and meditation are similarly related to focusing of awareness. When we learn to bring about this kind of concentration at will, we can be independent of external triggers for highs, whether drugs, sex, or mangoes.

Yoga philosophy says that one step in this process is constant self-reminding that the high comes from within, not from without — from the nervous system, not from the mango. Being at an early stage of this practice, I was furious to arrive in Panama and find only a few scrawny mangoes for sale. "It's too early," people told me, not at all impressed when I waved my arms and shouted that it was not too early in Costa Rica. I had a terrible premonition — correct, as it turned out — that I would get to Colombia and be told I was too late. It is a hard thing to break the mango habit by going cold turkey.

5

EATING CHILIES

TRYING TO IMAGINE India without red pepper is as difficult as trying to imagine Italy without tomatoes. Yet neither of these fruits was available to the Old World until Columbus brought them back from the Americas.

News of the New World's hot peppers traveled fast. In 1493 an historian, Peter Martyr, reported that Columbus had discovered peppers more pungent than those of Asia, and within a few years the plants themselves reached the Far East. They established themselves so well in Southeast Asia and India that some early botanists thought they were native there. Up to that time, the spice-loving peoples of the Orient had had to content themselves with black pepper, ginger, and mustard. Red pepper opened up whole new levels of hotness and is today indispensable in the cuisines of all of tropical Asia, western China, and Africa.

Technically, red pepper is not a pepper at all. It was named so because it is pungent, like black pepper, which is a member of the pepper family. Red pepper comes from the fruit of many varieties of the genus *Capsicum* in the potato or nightshade family. Our sweet green and red bell peppers are also capsicums. All capsicums are green when unripe, and all become yellow, orange, or red if allowed to ripen. The flavor and texture of the fruit change during ripening. For some purposes, crisp green pods are better; for others, the sweeter, softer red ones. Hot varieties of capsicum are called chilies. Cayenne is one type of chili, usually seen as a powder made from dried ripe pods.

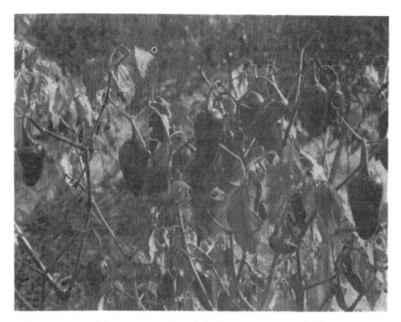

Jalapeños, one of the most popular of the hot peppers, are fairly pungent. In Mexican cuisine they are often pickled or cut up green, as a garnish. (Richard Schweid)

Chili is a truly American food. New World Indians might have been eating wild chilies 8000 years ago and were probably cultivating them as early as 5000 years ago. Chilies are among the oldest cultivated plants of the Americas. Under the influence of human planters, their wild progenitors assumed very diverse horticultural forms. In any open market in Mexico today, the traveler will see a bewildering array of chilies of all shapes, sizes, and degrees of pungency. The commonest varieties are named and used for specific purposes: The *jalapeño* is often pickled; the milder *ancho* is stuffed; the *poblano* is ground into *mole*, a seasoning mixture for stews that includes bitter chocolate and is derived from an ancient dish of chilies and chocolate reserved for Aztec royalty; the tiny, fiery *pequín* is ripened and dried for a powdered spice; and the even smaller and hotter *chiltepín*, still collected in the wild in desert regions of northern Mexico, is revered for its medicinal as well as culinary properties.

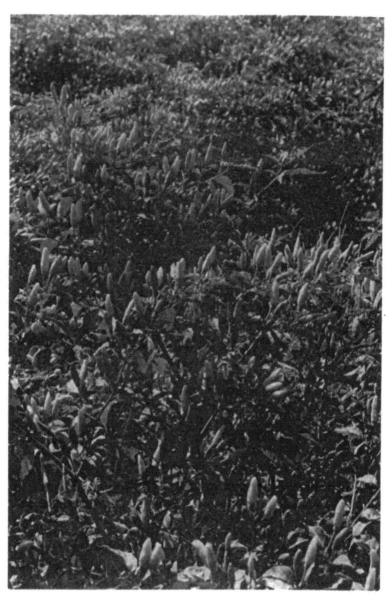

Tabasco peppers on Avery Island, Louisiana. This hot pepper was brought by the McIlhenny family from Mexico to Louisiana, where it is cultivated for Tabasco sauce. The sauce is a mash of red, ripe peppers, cured in salt, aged in wood, and later mixed with vinegar. (Richard Schweid)

Besides the many named varieties, there are dozens and dozens of nameless chilies, unknown beyond their localities of origin.

Chili eating in Mexico is a national pastime and constant source of wonder to tender-mouthed visitors from the North. As a rich source of vitamin C, richer than citrus, chili is a most important addition to the traditional peasant diet of tortillas and beans. But even a rugged Texan used to the hot chili con carne of the border regions may be stopped in his tracks by some of the peppers casually munched down by Mexican children as if they were gumdrops. I have a picture in mind of an Indian house I stayed in once in northeast Oaxaca, where a five-year-old girl delighted in nibbling on the hottest fresh chilies she could find, fanning her mouth with her hand between bites, and exclaiming over and over to me, *"Se pica, se pica"* ("It bites, it bites") with an expression of total rapture.

The word *capsicum* may derive from Latin *capsa,* "a box," suggesting the boxlike shape of the fruits of some varieties, but it may come also from Greek *kapto,* meaning "I bite." The latter seems more to the point. The biting quality of capsicum is due to the presence of capsaicin, a compound closely related to vanillin in its chemical structure. It is a very stable substance that persists through long cooking, drying, and aging, so that chilies retain their hotness well. The presence of capsaicin in the fruits is determined by a single dominant gene, so that if sweet peppers are crossed with hot ones, the progeny will all be hot. Incidentally, the maximum concentrations of this compound occur in the placenta, the whitish tissue to which the seeds are attached. Hot peppers may be tamed considerably by removing the placenta and seeds before adding them to other food.

The effect of capsaicin on the oral membranes is spectacular. A person uninitiated into the mysteries of chili eating who bites down on a really peppy capsicum pod may exhibit all the symptoms of furious rabies. It is difficult to convey to such a sufferer the truth that relief comes only of eating more chilies, but that is the case. Water makes the agony worse. Bread may be slightly helpful. But the only real help comes of plunging in and developing tolerance to the effect. Here we separate the chili lovers from the chili haters. There are those who believe that cayenne pepper is to be dispensed in barely visible pinches and Tabasco sauce in minuscule drops. I am not one of them. To me chilies are an inviting challenge, and I strive to master the art of eating them like a true son of the Americas. I have watched Mexicans cover a slice of fresh pineapple with powdered red chili. I have seen them eat whole pickled jalapeños between bites of sandwiches and cover tortillas with smoky, barbecued *chilpotle* peppers, so hot you expect them to eat through their containers. I have seen Mexican youths engage in chili-eating contests to extend their limits. I can tell by their expressions that all of these people are onto something good.

Now there must be a reason why so much of the world's population loves to eat chilies. Why should people willingly subject themselves to something that on first meeting seems so painful and irritating?

There is no question that capsicum can be irritating. Aerosol sprays of liquid capsicum have protected postmen from attacking dogs and city dwellers from muggers. Here is another American tradition: The Incas used liquid capsicum and the smoke of burning pods as agents of chemical warfare. Capsicum has been used as an agent of torture in both the New and Old Worlds. I have read that among the ancient Mayans it was customary to rub chili into the eyes of young girls caught glancing at men. If a girl were proved unchaste she had chili rubbed into her private parts as punishment. The smoke from burning chili pods is an effective fumigant; it will clear a room of human beings within seconds and of vermin in about an hour.

Although the irritation produced by chili is intense, it does not seem to do any damage. Inhabitants of Europe and temperate North America are inclined to look down upon chili eating as a nasty habit of the tropics, likely to be bad for the health and especially for the well-being of the stomach. But all herbalists regard capsicum as an excellent therapeutic agent, particularly beneficial for the stomach and entire digestive tract. Books on herbal medicine are unanimous on this point and recommend capsicum vigorously for many uses. For example, Jethro Kloss, author of the popular herbal, *Back to Eden,* writes of it:

> There is, perhaps, no other article which produces so powerful an impression on the animal frame that is so destitute of all injurious properties. [Capsicum] seems almost incapable of abuse, for however great the excitement produced by it, this stimulant prevents that excitement subsiding so suddenly as to induce any great derangement of the equilibrium of the circulation. It produces the most powerful impression on the surface yet never draws a blister; on the stomach, yet never weakens its tone. It is so diffusive in its character that it never produces any local lesion or induces permanent inflammation.*

Capsicum can be used topically in many ways. Poultices of it can be applied to relieve the pains of rheumatism and neuritis. Plasters of it may be more effective than mustard plasters for congestion of the chest or muscle pains. Thick pastes of red pepper can be applied directly to the tenderest skin without ill effect, say the books, although the sensation will be intense. Heavy sprinklings of chili in the socks may help cold toes and feet. I know many people who gargle with capsicum to treat sore throats and say it helps. Oil of capsicum will anesthetize and sterilize tooth cavities and may relieve toothache for months.

For internal use, powdered chili may be taken in hot water as a tea or swallowed in capsules. The dose, according to herbalists, is as much as one can tolerate. Large doses of red pepper are recommended for the treatment of alcoholic gastritis and ulcers, a prescription that would certainly appall the average internist. It is a sensible remedy because chili brings a great deal of blood to the surface of mucous membranes, and increased blood supply should promote healing. Taken internally, chili is said to purify the blood, tone the liver, and clear the respiratory tract.

---

* (New York: Beneficial Books, 1971), p. 217.

The true chili lover may be aware of these medicinal properties, but the motive for passion lies elsewhere. It is the immediate effect of capsicum in the mouth that endears it to so many people — and repels so many others. A large dose of chili causes an intense sensation of burning that spreads up the nose, producing nasal secretion and tearing from the eyes. It is an excellent way to clear the sinuses. The sensation in the mouth may become so strong that one cannot think about anything else for a few minutes. Capsicum also stimulates the flow of perspiration, an effect that may be welcome in a hot climate. Together these actions give a proper rush, and it is this rush that the chili lover seeks.

Now, the experience of a chili lover is different from that of a chili hater. The chili hater suffers actual pain and goes to great lengths to combat the sensation in his mouth before trying another bite. Finally, after repeated attempts, all equally painful, he excuses himself, saying he is not a masochist. Neither, of course, is the chili lover. He knows that pain can be transformed into a friendly sensation whose strength can go into making him high. The secret of this trick lies in perceiving that the sensation follows the form of a wave: It builds to a terrifying peak, then subsides, leaving the body completely unharmed. Chili eating is painful when you have to go from the trough of the wave to the crest over and over again. Familiarity with the sensation makes it possible to eat chili at a rate that keeps the intensity constant. One is then able to glide along on the strong stimulation, experiencing it as something between pleasure and pain that enforces concentration and brings about a high state of consciousness. This technique might be called "mouth surfing."

With practice, faith, and the frequent company of capsicum lovers, one can develop quickly into a first-rate chili eater, learning to appreciate the more pungent varieties in ever-increasing doses. "But that is an addiction," the chili hater will exclaim with contempt. I suppose it is possible to become as dependent on chilies as on anything else that can provide a high. Santha Rama Rau, in her book, *The Cooking of India*, recounts the story of

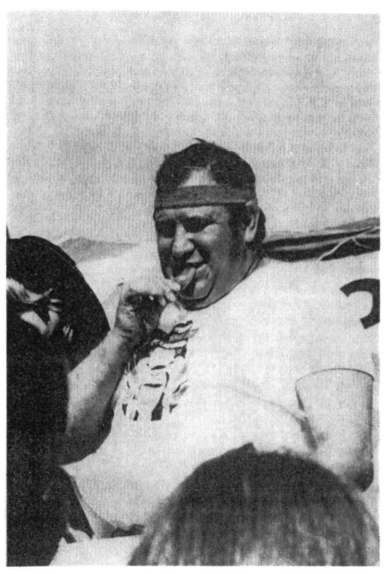

Contestant in a jalapeño-eating contest in New Mexico. Such events are highlights of chili festivals in New Mexico, where most hot peppers are grown in the United States. To win the contest, not only must you eat the largest number of jalapeños but you must refrain from spluttering, choking, or belching, all of which lead to disqualification. (Courtesy International Connoisseurs of Red and Green Chile, Las Cruces, New Mexico)

an Indian friend who was traveling from India to the United States. She stopped off at the London airport, and while there she met a girl from Andhra in South India. The girl was on her way to the States to join her husband, a graduate student at the University of Pittsburgh. She had been sick for two days at the airport hotel with an upset stomach, brought on, she explained, by the blandness of the food. Everything was like eating chalk, she said. She ordered an omelet for breakfast and complained that it had no taste. My friend asked the waiter to bring a bottle of Tabasco in a hurry, and poured three quarters of it on the omelet. That was better, the girl said, but it still was not hot enough. So my friend asked the waiter for some peppers. He brought a bottle, and she dumped fourteen to sixteen red-hot South American peppers on top of the omelet. The girl's eyes lit up when she tasted it. "Ah, Bhenji (sister)," she said with relief, "Now I have come to life!" *

I find that my desire to eat chili is cyclic. For a week or so I may eat it three times a day, adding it with pleasure to many dishes and enjoying a really intense chili rush at least once each day. Then I will go without it for a while. Even when I am eating it in quantity, my enjoyment of bland foods is undiminished. When I start in again I do not have to go through a period of adaptation. My chili tolerance now seems to be permanent.

Just as I was helped in learning to be a chili lover by spending time around masters of the art, I am now able to help others. I have guided several people from the initial stages of mouth burning to intermediate and advanced levels of chili eating and am always gratified to watch them discover the joys of this practice and marvel at their newfound abilities. It is always uplifting to conquer something that once seemed unattainable. It is especially meaningful to see that by a change of mental attitude, perseverance, and openness to new experience something that previously appeared painful and injurious can become pleasureful and beneficial.

* (New York: Time-Life Books, 1969), p. 95.

6

A GOOD FIT

HAVE YOU EVER laughed so hard that tears streamed down your face and you found yourself collapsed on the floor, almost unable to breathe? How did you feel immediately afterward? Cleaned out? Invigorated? Healthy? High? Although there is considerable social pressure against losing control of oneself in such a flamboyant way, most people who experience true fits of laughter feel very good indeed when they recover their composure. We have all heard that "laughter is the best medicine." That might be true and might have a special neurological basis.

I am interested here not in guffaws or chuckles, which are simply learned vocalizations, but in uncontrollable spasms of laughter — the kind that lead after several minutes to loss of upright posture, paralysis of the diaphragm (accounting for the inability to speak or breathe and the pain in the abdomen), and copious production of tears.

When I was growing up in Philadelphia, my father's mother, Mayme, lived with us for a time. She was subject to fits of what we called the "giggles" (a great understatement), and it was my impish pleasure to help set them off whenever I could. My grandmother seldom drank alcohol, but at family dinner parties she liked to have an after-dinner Alexander; apparently the gin in this drink was the priming agent. At least, at a certain point after imbibing her Alexander, Mayme was highly susceptible to spectacular laughing fits that could be brought on by the telling of jokes, by the laughing of others, or (my specialty) by surreptitious tickling. When my grandmother was "giggling," as we politely called it, any dinner party would grind to a halt, and the guests would sit in awkward silence while Mayme laughed herself out, usually in ten minutes. When she was finished, her face would be flushed and wet with tears, she would breathe in short gasps, and would gradually return to normal consciousness. The family dinner would resume, and my grandmother's performance would never be mentioned. I, for one, got a terrific contact high from it.

I have always suspected that Mayme was onto a good thing, and I am happy to have inherited in some degree the ability to abandon myself to hysterical laughter. It feels that good. Only recently have I bothered to wonder why it is good to laugh till you cry.

Not much information is available on the physiology of laughter. But something is known about tear production (lacrimation). That might be a convenient starting point.

All on their own, continuously, and independently of their nerve supplies, the lacrimal glands produce a certain amount of tears to keep the surface of the eye moist. This is called basic secretion. A second kind of lacrimation is in response to certain drugs called secretogogues that stimulate the glands directly when dropped into the eye. A third kind is reflex tearing, in response to strong stimulation of the optic nerve (bright light) or olfactory nerve (red pepper), or in response to irritation of the eyeball itself (smoke). In all of these cases, the offending stimulus is carried to the brain by sensory nerves, eventually to reach and trigger a group of cells called the lacrimal nucleus. The nerve fibers originating in this nucleus carry the outgoing impulse to the tear glands, making them secrete. These outgoing nerves are part of the parasympathetic division of the autonomic, or "involuntary," nervous system.

Now, the lacrimal nucleus is in a part of the brainstem called the pons. The brainstem is a group of midline structures connecting the cerebral hemispheres to the spinal cord. The pons is midway along it, lying between the lowest brainstem structure, the medulla, and the midbrain higher up. Many of the involuntary functions of our bodies have their controlling centers in the brainstem, and many of the most important parasympathetic nerves originate here. The brainstem is thus a locus of much of our unconscious mental activity, just as the cerebral hemispheres are the seat of our conscious mental life. The brainstem is a physical connection between the hemispheres and the spinal cord; it may also be thought of as a connection between mind and body.

I have mentioned three types of tearing. There is a fourth, known as psychogenic tearing, and it seems to be peculiar to humans. Psychogenic tearing is tearing that accompanies emotional states: crying in joy or pain or sorrow, and laughing. It is mind-caused lacrimation and is mediated in the same way as reflex tearing — that is, from the lacrimal nucleus to the glands via parasympathetic fibers — but the causative stimulus originates in the mind (presumably in the cortex of the cerebral hemispheres) rather than in the periphery of the body. Animals do not show psychogenic tearing; the humor of laughing hyenas is quite dry. Nor do newborn infants have it. Most babies do not cry emotional tears until they are a month old.

The discovery of anything unique to humans is important as a clue to what we are, especially if it is a phenomenon that sheds light on the relationships between our minds and bodies. I have written often that a key to health of mind and body is integration of conscious and unconscious activity. The more open and functioning are the channels between the day mind and the night mind, the more we can consciously receive and benefit from the influences that come to us through the unconscious. At the same time, we can exert beneficial effects on our bodies by means of these same channels — as in the control of violent emotional states by the conscious regulation of breathing. A condition of open communication between the conscious and unconscious obtains whenever the observing ego gets out of the way. In a fit of laughter there is no ego — no censorship of messages flowing back and forth in the brain. What strikes the mind funny simultaneously sets off a self-perpetuating cycle of nervous discharges in the brainstem. Tearing is one manifestation of this exercise of the autonomic system. The diaphragmatic spasms are another. Mind and body are laughing together; the channels are wide open.

Loss of upright posture is further evidence that in a fit of laughter the cerebral cortex is not maintaining its usual hold on brain function. I say this because it occurs in other conditions where it is clearly associated with suspension of cortical activity. Grand mal epilepsy — "falling sickness" — is an example. Another is a rare ailment called cataplexy, whose symptoms are discrete attacks of loss of upright posture, usually triggered by spontaneous emotion, especially laughter. It is reasonable to conclude that when a laughing fit proceeds to the point of dropping to the floor, there is a higher-than-usual ratio of brainstem versus cortical activity — of unconscious versus conscious determination of experience.

Not surprisingly, the result is a high. Exhaustion may follow, too, but it is the exhaustion of a feat accomplished, of work well done. I cannot imagine that the effect on the body is anything but that of an invigorating tonic and cleanser. In fact, I am tempted to base an entire system of medical practice on the induction of laughing fits in patients.

Of course, painful stimuli will produce flows of tears, too, and, no doubt, good solid crys are also cathartic and beneficial. In *The Naked Ape*, Desmond Morris writes: ". . . it is important to realize how similar crying and laughing are, as response patterns. Their moods are so different that we tend to overlook this . . . It appears that the laughing response evolved out of the crying one . . . ."*

In certain kinds of modern psychotherapy, such as group encounter, great value is placed on breaking down the defenses of participants. If people are reduced to tears, for instance, the encounter is successful. These tears may be therapeutic. But encouraging reintegration of the personality afterward is much more difficult than breaking down de-

---

* (New York: McGraw-Hill, 1967), p. 116.

fenses, and the encounter method is sometimes not successful with it.

An interesting medical application of crying is suggested by the Reverend Robert Alexander, bishop, founder, and director of The Temple of Man in Venice, California. He wrote me recently:

> For many years now, perhaps thirty in all, I have been trying to convince people that the explanation of the common cold lies in understanding that the symptoms are caused by the uncried tears of man — tears not expressed through normal grief-releasing mechanisms. Perhaps, what with the Wailing Wall of the Ancients in good wailing order, we, too, could relieve ourselves of this pesky disorder with nothing more than a good honest cry.

Perhaps so. But other things being equal, I would rather laugh my way to health and enlightenment than weep it, and I wonder how to turn more people on to the value of outrageous laughter.

The relationship of drugs to laughter is not direct, although three drugs are associated with it. Those three are alcohol, marijuana, and nitrous oxide, also known as laughing gas. Hilarity is often a symptom of the early stages of alcoholic inebriation, especially in groups. Larger doses of alcohol more commonly produce boisterousness or morose withdrawal. Nitrous oxide, which has a pharmacological effect similar to alcohol but is a much less toxic drug, also can cause hilarious laughter at low doses, particularly in groups. Higher doses, taken in less convivial settings, are more often associated with states of deep introspective reverie and philosophic or mystic insights that evaporate almost as soon as one stops breathing the gas. Marijuana, a different sort of drug, also facilitates laughter — again, more in group settings where participants are set to laugh.

Laughing fits seem correlated with drug effects only to the extent that the drugs allow for a moderate degree of social disinhibition. There is no laugh center in the brain that is stimulated by alcohol, marijuana, and laughing gas. Rather, the mild effects of these drugs at low-dose ranges in appropriate settings provide excuses for people to lose control of themselves. My grandmother would never allow herself to have the giggles most of the time. The after-dinner Alexander became a ritual excuse that was tolerated by her relatives, all of whom, I am sure, wanted to be laughing along with her but could not let themselves go.

Any situation encouraging social disinhibition favors laughing fits. Perhaps the best trigger of all is the sight of someone else doing it, for laughing, like yawning, is highly contagious. A really good laugher in the right setting can get a lot of other people to join in. Done ritually and regularly, group laughing fits could serve as the basis for a new system of psychotherapy or even a new religion. Wouldn't that be nice?

7

MUSHROOMS I

GORDON WASSON, who rediscovered the ritual use of psychedelic mushrooms in Mexico, wrote some years ago that people can be divided into mycophiles and mycophobes — mushroom lovers and mushroom haters.* There seems to be no middle ground. To some individuals and to some entire cultures, mushrooms are not fit for human consumption, and the idea of eating them is disgusting. This deeply felt revulsion might be linked with fear of being poisoned. Stories of mushroom poisonings evoke images of ghastly deaths, and I know some persons who shun even cultivated mushrooms in the fear that they might really be "toadstools."

Wasson explains mycophobia as fear of the mysteries to which certain mushrooms give access. Apparently, from remote times, some species have been used ritually, and often secretly, to put initiates into other states of consciousness and other dimensions of experience. Possibly the *soma* of the ancient Aryans was *Amanita muscaria*, the bright red Fly Agaric. Probably the potion drunk at the Eleusinian mysteries in ancient Greece was a decoction of a psychoactive fungus.† Certainly, to the rational, intellectual, ego-centered side of human consciousness, such mysteries and the keys of access to them are things to be feared.

* R. Gordon Wasson and Valentina P. Wasson, *Mushrooms, Russia and History* (New York: Pantheon Books, 1957).
† See R. Gordon Wasson, Carl A. P. Ruck, and Albert Hofmann, *The Road to Eleusis: Unveiling the Secret of the Mysteries* (New York: Harcourt Brace Jovanovich, 1978).

I am a long-time mycophile. To me, mushrooms are strangely beautiful, fascinating, delicious. I prefer wild ones to cultivated ones and find myself curious to sample some of the species that books call poisonous. To me, fear of toadstools looks irrational. The percentage of mushrooms that are deadly is very small, and the deadly species can easily be learned and avoided. As for some of the other "poisonous" ones — well, one man's toxin is another man's psychedelic. But I readily admit that mushrooms are strange, magical, and, therefore, dangerous.

They are, above all, perfect symbols of the "other" side of consciousness, of what Robert Ornstein in his book, *The Psychology of Consciousness*, calls the "night" side, the nonordinary mode of the dreamer, the visionary, the artist, the intuitive thinker. Ornstein, a psychologist interested both in neurology and esoteric systems of mind development, presents evidence that the two hemispheres of the brain serve very different functions. One is the locus of language, of linear thought, of masculine or "day" consciousness; the other is the locus of nonlinear, nonrational, feminine, receptive, intuitional consciousness. Of meditation, Ornstein writes: "[It] . . . is a technique for turning down the brilliance of the day, so that everpresent and subtle sources of energy can be perceived within. It constitutes a deliberate attempt to separate oneself for a short period from the flow of daily life, and to 'turn off' the active mode of normal consciousness, in order to enter the complementary mode of 'darkness' and receptivity."*

What we call *a* mushroom is the fruiting body of a form of life that exists in the soil as a vast network of microscopic cellular threads, invisible to the naked eye except in mass. The fruiting body is a gigantic, compact aggregation of these threads, the result of rapid cell division and growth. Some mushrooms can develop in several hours after a soaking rain. It is this character of springing up full-grown in all of their strange beauty that makes mushrooms such potent

*(San Francisco: Freeman, 1972), p. 107.

symbols of the workings of our unconscious minds. Intu-itions, flashes of insight, mystical raptures all burst into or-dinary consciousness in all their vividness from the dark, in-visible substratum of mind that exists below and within the daylight world of everyday. Like mushrooms, they cannot long exist in the sun but must be taken advantage of as soon as they appear.

Mushrooms lack chlorophyll, so they cannot derive energy directly from the sun but must feed on live or dead organic matter. In nature they are vital intermediaries in the life cycle: They dismantle complicated organic structures to simplest constituents that can be used again to build the material shells of living things. Their fruiting bodies are works of great complexity compared to the simple strands of cells woven through the soil below.

It is hard to look at certain mushrooms without being struck by their phallic shape. Some species, the stinkhorns in particular, are so flagrant in this resemblance that they carry the word *phallus* in their botanical names. Here is another meaningful correspondence: The form of the mush-room is homologous with the form of a part of the human body that has very direct connections to the night side of the mind.

So it is not surprising that mushrooms are associated with mysteries, with flights of the soul from the body, and with death itself.* For all of these experiences are rooted in un-conscious mental activity.

I have suggested that some mushrooms called poisonous in books might equally well be called psychedelic. All psy-chedelics are intoxicants — that is, poisons. The decision to use a positively or negatively loaded term has nothing to do with the reality of the thing itself. *Amanita muscaria* is an example. It is called the "Fly Agaric" (*agaric* is another word for "mushroom") because an infusion of it in milk was set out in olden times to kill houseflies. Nearly all books call

---

* The mushroom cloud is an archetypal symbol of death for the twentieth century.

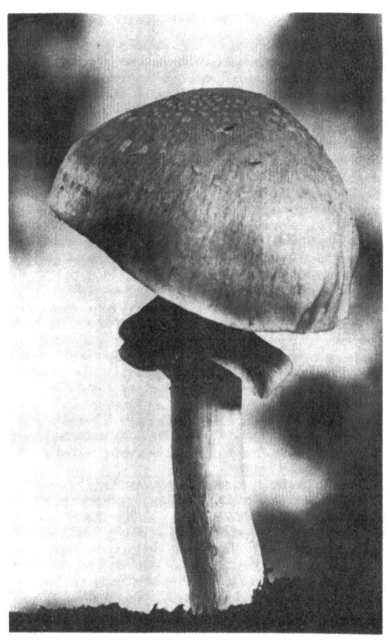

The San Isidro mushroom, *Psilocybe cubensis*. (Bob Harris)

Amanita muscaria dangerous, if not deadly, probably because it is a relative of a much more dangerous mushroom, *Amanita phalloides*, the Death Cup. Yet there is no question that *A. muscaria* can transport people, quite safely, to realms of powerful, nonordinary experience. At the present time, many people in northern California are using it to take themselves on such trips, some by drinking infusions of it in milk.

A simple explanation of this disparity in the reported effects of the Fly Agaric in man is that people are differently set to interpret effects of this sort. *Amanita muscaria* does not kill, but it does make the body feel very unusual. This strong but neutral change may be interpreted in one of two ways: as a negative, outside force operating against the ego — that is, as sickness or intoxication — or as an opportunity to withdraw attention from ordinary things and pay attention to strange ones — that is, as an altered state of consciousness or high.

In other words, there is no line between poisonous and psychedelic mushrooms. Mushrooms are a pharmacological continuum, from the white cultivated variety that has no action as a drug to species like the Death Cup that can easily kill. If one likes to get high by eating mushrooms, he can choose species over a wide range of toxicity.

In Latin America I had a number of experiences with psychedelic-poisonous mushrooms.

*

Probably the best mushrooms to use as psychedelics are those containing psilocybin, a drug that is relatively gentle on the physical organism yet strongly capable of inducing visionary experience. A number of species contain this substance, many in the genus *Psilocybe*, for which it is named. Of the several kinds of psilocybin mushrooms available in Mexico, where their ritual consumption is an old Indian tradition, I tried only one: the species *Psilocybe* (or *Stropharia*) *cubensis*, known colloquially as San Isidro.

This mushroom grows widely throughout tropical and

subtropical America. It has a light tan cap, darker at the center; dark gills; and a blackish veil around the stem. Any part of it that is bruised turns blue within minutes. It grows in open cow pastures at the edges of clumps of cow manure, and its size is variable. I have seen caps up to a foot in diameter. Because its appearance and growth habits are so characteristic, one can easily learn to distinguish it and collect it.

The San Isidro mushroom is eaten by Mazatec and other Indians in the Sierra Mazateca in the northeastern corner of the Mexican state of Oaxaca and by many outsiders who come to the area to "do mushrooms." It is available during the rainy season from May to September and also at any time rain falls during the rest of the year. I arrived in Huáutla de Jiménez, the main town of the area, just after a fortuitous out-of-season downpour at the end of January 1972 and so was able to obtain and eat a quantity of San Isidro mushrooms.

Huáutla is where Gordon Wasson, over twenty years ago, met Maria Sabina, a priestess who introduced him to the ceremonial use of *hongos* — sacred mushrooms. Today, Maria Sabina lives mostly in seclusion on a ridge outside the town but offers to sell autographed pictures of herself to visitors. The Indians of the area, who once guarded their secret rites zealously from outsiders, now embroider shirts with mushroom motifs and phrases like "Magic Mushroom" and "Peace and Love" in English, for sale in the Oaxaca city market.

Starting in the late 1960s, Huáutla was flooded by thousands of mushroom-seeking hippies from Mexico, the United States, and Europe. On several occasions, government troops were sent in to clear the hippies out. There were ugly confrontations between armed soldiers and defenseless seekers of highs. In 1972 a sullen mood hung over the Sierra Mazateca. Outsiders were not welcome. Occasional longhairs wandered in, and by paying "voluntary" donations to the local school, could get permits from civil authorities to hang around and try for mushrooms. They were sometimes chased out by the military.

I had the good fortune to be taken into the house of Julieta, a *curandera* (healer) who lives in a tiny village near Huáutla and who uses mushrooms in religious services and medical curings. But the village council was not happy with my presence and told me I would be put in jail if I stayed beyond sunset. After much arguing (not easy, since almost no one spoke Spanish), I wangled a twenty-four-hour permit to stay, and Julieta said she would keep me hidden away in her kitchen to minimize my visibility. Because her house was directly across the street from the little town hall, I was constantly aware of the tension surrounding my presence and of the need for secrecy in all things to do with the mushrooms.

The Sierra Mazateca is a breathtakingly beautiful area of Mexico, with steep green peaks, rushing rivers, and hillsides of coffee and banana trees. The little villages are clustered on the very tops of the mountains so that going from one to another means long and difficult descents and ascents over rough roads. From Julieta's house one could see Huáutla on a neighboring peak and other settlements in the distance — a splendid vista. The house itself had three rooms: a tiny kitchen; a large, sparsely furnished living room; and a bedroom, where eight or nine persons slept at night. Julieta was the head of the household, and her husband seemed to defer to her in all important matters. They had five children. A young girl who tended the house also lived with them.

From morning to night, a constant stream of patients came to be treated by Julieta, to chat, to drink coffee. Mothers with sick babies, children with bad cuts, grownups with stomach trouble all wandered in, stayed for minutes or hours, got their medicine, and left. Julieta had a garden of medicinal herbs growing in back of her house. She talked much about hongos as the *gran remedio* that cured all ills, but in the everyday situations that confronted her she relied on modern drugs. A table in the living room was heaped with antibiotics and other chemicals, mostly in injectable forms. Like many curanderas in Mexico, Julieta is skilled in giving injections, and most patients who come to her want injections, even of drugs that can just as well be given by mouth. The Mazatecs have come to see injection as a magical technique, more magical than their traditional practices. Antibiotics and other powerful drugs (many of them dangerous, in my view) are widely available without prescription in Latin America and wind up in the hands of nonprofessional therapists like Julieta. Although I disagree with her methods of treatment, I must say that she knew what she was doing and that she inspired faith and confidence in people who had no one else to turn to when they were sick. There seemed to be a lot of sickness in and around Huáutla, fostered by inbreeding in an area long isolated from the outside by difficult mountains. Illness is also encouraged by the damp chill that permeates the region whenever clouds block out the tropical sun.

Shortly before my arrival, Julieta had picked a bunch of San Isidro mushrooms. They were obviously meant for me, she said, although I had arrived out of the blue with no forewarning. The mushrooms were wrapped in a sheet of newspaper, hidden in the bedroom, waiting for the right moment to be used. That moment came after midnight on the night after my arrival, which was also the night of the full moon in January, after the last patient had gone home, the children had been put to bed, and the house boarded up for the night. Julieta, her husband, the servant girl, and I gathered in the kitchen by candlelight. Julieta unpacked a bag of paraphernalia for the ceremony while her husband set up a small altar on a low table. The centerpiece of the altar was a framed portrait of San Isidro.

San Isidro is the patron saint of agricultural workers and a popular household saint throughout Mexico. Julieta explained that he was her husband's patron saint and that she used him to preside over her mushroom ceremony. It was just "coincidence" that the variety of mushroom we were going to use also bore his name. The standard depiction of San Isidro is striking: In the midst of a beautiful pastoral scene, an obviously holy man in brown robes kneels in prayer beside a cart and oxen, looking up to heaven. Above, through an opening in the sky, psychedelic rays pour down upon him from some other dimension. Julieta told me to concentrate on the picture while she got things ready.

In front of the altar was a small charcoal fire. On it Julieta burned incense — *copal* (a resin related to frankincense) and *palo santo* (an aromatic wood). She sat beside me on a woven mat, purifying her hands and face in the fragrant smoke while whispering prayers. She asked me to cleanse myself in the smoke in the same way. Then she took up the mushrooms in the sheet of newspaper, studied them for a long time, picking up one and then another, all the time praying and wafting incense smoke over herself. The mushrooms were about two days old by now, somewhat wrinkled and dry, with many larvae and little winged insects crawling over them. Julieta bathed them in the smoke, praying more fervently. Her husband and the servant girl retired several paces to a darker area of the kitchen and waited in silence.

When the incense was consumed, Julieta took a small dried chili pod and placed it on the glowing charcoal. She passed the mushrooms through the acrid smoke that went up from the chili, and instantly the larvae and insects crawled out of the mushrooms and died on the newspaper. The chili was removed and more copal put in its place.

Now the time had come. With great deliberation, Julieta took the two largest mushrooms (three-inch caps), arranged them on a little dish, and handed the dish to me. She told me the mushrooms were like the Eucharist and that taking them inside me would enable me to participate in the mystery of the service. Then she smiled sweetly and asked me where my parents were and whether it was all right with them that I was doing this. I told her they were in Philadelphia and trusted me. She seemed satisfied and told me to eat the mushrooms.

I began chewing the cap of the larger mushroom. It was a bit dry and surprisingly tasty: a strong, penetrating, wild mushroom flavor that became more intense as I chewed. I had not anticipated how good these things would be to eat.

So many Indian drugs I have tried are intensely bitter, replete with warnings to the senses that they are not supposed to be eaten. But here was something delicious. Before I knew it, I had finished both, stems and all. Julieta now prepared another dish, this time with seven or eight smaller mushrooms. She bathed them in incense, praying as before, and handed the dish to me. I ate them one by one, chewing thoroughly. This operation was repeated two more times, so that I ate a total of about twenty smaller mushrooms. Julieta then fed several mushrooms to her husband and to the servant girl, asking them first to wash their hands and faces in the scented smoke and praying over them quietly as they ate. She then told me to sit still while she made sure all the children were asleep.

It must have been one in the morning. Through a crack in the kitchen window I could see that the lights of the town hall were still burning. Doubtless, the council was still debating whether or not to put the intrusive gringo in jail. But in back of the house, all was dark: the eerie blackness of the Sierra Mazateca and now the brilliant splendor of a full moon, high over the mountains in a cloudless sky. I sat watching San Isidro in the flickering candlelight, feeling extraordinarily content and well. Julieta's husband leaned over from time to time, asking if I was all right and assuring me that his wife would soon be back. I told him I was fine.

By the time Julieta reappeared, I was just beginning to feel unusual. The effect of the mushrooms was very gentle, definite, and progressive, beginning as a sensation of lightness and well-being. Julieta placed more incense on the charcoal. Now her husband and the servant girl left us alone. I was kneeling in front of the little altar; Julieta knelt to one side, praying continuously to San Isidro and other intercessors to help me in my life's work. She asked me to repeat the Lord's Prayer three times. I began to see color hallucinations — pastel spots and gentle undulations of surfaces — all delightful.

My recollection is that we prayed together for some time during the peak of the effect of the mushrooms, probably from forty-five minutes to an hour and a half after I had eaten them. I felt fresh, alert, healthy, and cleansed. Then, the formal part of the service over, Julieta and I chatted for a long while about personal matters. She communicated to me much of her own vitality, optimism, and goodness of spirit, leaving me elated and more confident in my own abilities and powers. Finally (it was now quite late), she told me to go outside and "learn from the moon." She said she had to go to bed and that I should stay up as long as I wanted and then sleep late the next day.

Outside, the night was magnificent. I felt privileged to have arrived at such a spot on such a night, feeling the way I did. The mushrooms were still strongly working on me. I could taste them more powerfully than ever, and the taste seemed to be diffused throughout my body, making me feel in a very real way that the spirit of the mushrooms had entered into me. I recalled Wasson's suggestion that the word "bemushroomed" would be a good term for this state. I was certainly bemushroomed.

I gazed at the moon and the landscape for perhaps an hour, then spent some more time with San Isidro in the kitchen. He, too, seemed bemushroomed out there in the field with all those heavenly rays raining down upon him. Then, after another interval, I went back outside. But now it was much darker, and a great many stars were out, whereas only a few had been visible before. I could not find the moon at first. Then I saw it, low over the western mountains: a crescent of silver along a dull gold disk. It was being eclipsed. I waited, breathless, as the eclipse progressed to totality — an unexpected, wonderful spectacle. The stillness of the night was complete; I doubt that very many people were awake to see the show in the sky.

Then the moon began to set behind the mountains, still in eclipse, and I felt tired for the first time. I went back inside, said good-night to San Isidro, blew out the candles, crawled into my sleeping bag, and fell asleep quickly.

In the morning, I awoke refreshed, feeling better than I had in a long time, and went off for a day in Huáutla of shopping and negotiating with the military authorities. (The council in Julieta's village was making more threats of jail-ing me, and I wanted some sort of safe-conduct pass.) When I got back, Julieta told me there were some mushrooms left over and that I might as well finish them that night. I really did not want to since I had just had a perfect mushroom experience, but instead of telling her that, I agreed. So that night we repeated the service with incense, prayers, and San Isidro, and then Julieta went to bed. But everything was different. A heavy bank of fog and cloud closed in, the temperature dropped, and suddenly nearly everyone in the house was sick. There was much crying and coughing from the bedroom, and I began feeling unwell, too. A great sense of depression and isolation came over me. I could not get to sleep. The mushrooms seemed to be working against me, not with me, and I felt far away from where I was suppose to be.

Toward dawn, still awake, I began to understand that this experience, too, was part of the lesson: that mushrooms, like other agents of psychedelic experience, must be used in a proper context, that their magic is strong but neutral and can produce evil as well as good. To take them just because they are available, when the time is not right, is a mistake. The negative experience of this second night did not in any way detract from the goodness of the first night. If anything, it made me more aware of the value of that experience and more eager to retain it and use it in my life. I hoped that I would be able to be bemushroomed again, but I resolved to be patient until the right moment came.

At the first light of dawn, I got up and packed my things. We had decided it would be best for me to leave before the sun was up so that I could be out of the clutches of those officials who wanted no outsiders on their mountaintop. I said good-bye gratefully to Julieta and started down the mountain toward the world outside.

*

An interesting piece of news from South America was the discovery of psilocybin mushrooms in Colombia in the late 1960s. Some species, especially *Psilocybe cubensis*, had been reported outside Mexico, but it was assumed that their use was confined to Oaxaca and neighboring territories. About 1967, stories began to reach the United States that students in Colombia were getting high by eating mushrooms.

Colombia is a sort of cornucopia of psychoactive plants. In addition to producing a multitude of exotic Amazonian drugs, like yagé, it is the main source of potent marijuana in western South America and a large coca producer as well. Now, it seems, it is a second home for psilocybin mushrooms. *Psilocybe cubensis*, the San Isidro of Mexico, has established itself in many parts of the country, and many people consume it. There is no tradition for use of mushrooms as intoxicants by South American Indians, so that knowledge of use of this species must have come from outside. Quite probably it came by way of hippies — North American, South American, or European — who knew the mushroom from the Huáutla area of Oaxaca and recognized it in Colombia. In some cases, these people have recently introduced Colombian Indians to the drug, the reverse of the usual order of things.

Many stories about *Psilocybe cubensis* circulate among travelers in Colombia. One is that it grows wherever volcanoes, fireflies, and avocadoes occur together. Another is that it follows Brahma cattle, which were imported into South America in this century because of their resistance to heat. But it seems to be growing all over the place without regard to any particular conditions and even fruits in great abundance in central Florida and along the Gulf Coast of the United States, where volcanoes, at least for the moment, are not much in evidence.

Nearly every major Colombian city has a mushroom field not far from it. There is a big one at La Miel ("Honey"), reachable by bus, milk truck, and footpath from Bogotá; one in the hills above Medellín; another just at the edge of Cali. After rains, when the hongos are plentiful, these fields are full of young people picking and eating the magic plants. The mushrooms are growing all through the fertile Cauca Valley and in the Amazon basin as well. Other species, including some psilocybes previously known only in Mexico, are turning up, too — one of them right in the streets of

Bogotá. Yet so far, in South America they have not been seen outside of Colombia. For example, no one is finding them in Ecuador,* Peru, or Venezuela.

Because Colombia has such a concentration of drug plants and because it is also the easiest place in South America to reach from the United States, great numbers of North Americans come to sample the fruits of the land. Few of them seem to be disappointed with the mushrooms. I heard almost no stories of bad trips. Few persons get sick on mushrooms, and few have anything but good words to say about them. They are talked about with a kind of respect that one does not often hear from long-time users of many drugs.

I first ate Colombian mushrooms outside Cali in an idyllically beautiful field with clumps of woods, a clear river, and enormous, gray, hump-backed Brahma cows lying peacefully in the bright green grass. It was the beginning of the dry season, but there were enough hongos to bemushroom a group of us, and we ate them as we found them. To eat them fresh from the ground was a great treat to the senses.

We sat in the grass, about ten of us, and let the mushrooms transport us to a realm of calm good feeling in which we drank in the beauty of the setting. There were color visions, as I had experienced before with San Isidro in Mexico. In Mexico I had eaten the mushrooms late at night, in darkness and secrecy, in the very shadow of menacing police authority. Now it was broad daylight, in open country, with no one around but friendly fellow travelers. In Mexico I had felt like an early Christian pursuing the sacrament in a catacomb, wary for the approach of Roman legions; here everything was aboveground and open. The Indians of the Sierra Mazateca say that mushrooms should not be eaten in daytime, that they must be eaten at night. Yet here we were in full daylight having a wonderful time. In general, I prefer to take psychedelic substances in the daytime, when their stimulating energies are more in harmony

---

Psilocybe cubensis now grows in quantity in northern Ecuador, where it is probably a recent introduction.

with the rhythms of my body. I feel that way about mushrooms, too. Is it possible, I wondered, that the Indian habit of eating mushrooms at night is not so traditional as it seems but dates back only to the arrival of the Spanish and persecutions of native rites by the church?

After several hours, we wandered back through the imperturbable Brahma giants, across the river, and to the road where we had left our truck. Another nice thing about the mushrooms is that they wear off, gently, after four to six hours — a more convenient duration of action than the twelve-hour trips of LSD, peyote, mescaline, and MDA. We had some extra mushrooms still with us, and these we dried for later use. Some days later, on the deserted shore of a lake in the eastern Andes, near the border of Ecuador, a few of us shared these dried mushrooms and again felt their magic. Though they still tasted good, it was not as pleasant to eat them this way as fresh.

*

I believe strongly that psychedelics merely trigger or release certain experiences that originate in the human nervous system and that one can learn to have these experiences without taking drugs. I believe also that psychedelic substances are useful in certain people at certain times. For example, when used properly they have great potential for bringing about medical as well as psychological cures of morbid conditions. Of the psychedelics I am familiar with, few approach mushrooms in overall desirable qualities, such as ease of consumption, lack of toxicity, and manageability of effects.

At the same time, I must caution that the abrupt onset of major alterations in perception can easily cause panic reactions, especially in people who take the mushrooms casually in poor circumstances, rather than ceremonially. By standardizing set and setting, ritual and ceremony work to minimize the potential of drugs to cause negative experiences. Mushrooms certainly have that potential and must be used with due respect.

8

MUSHROOMS II

THE FIRST TIME I crossed the Oregon Cascades was in October 1971 when I was on my way to Mexico. I could scarcely believe the exuberance of fungal growth I saw in those mountains. I decided to come back one day to study mushrooms seriously. In October 1973 I kept that promise when I arrived in Eugene at the height of the fall season.

While crossing the country from New York, I read a number of mushroom handbooks to acquaint myself with the species I was likely to encounter. The one that particularly caught my fancy was the Chanterelle (*Cantharellus cibarius*), a large, fleshy, yellow-orange mushroom that grows abundantly in the fall in the Douglas Fir forests of the Pacific Northwest. It is a prized delicacy, hunted down enthusiastically by all true mycophiles. I had tried canned Chanterelles a few times (the United States imports them from France and Germany), but knew that was hardly a substitute for eating them fresh.

I got to Eugene on a Saturday afternoon, in time to go mushrooming with friends. Tim and Jane handed me a plastic bucket and a sharp knife and drove me to a nearby pasture.

Meadow Mushrooms (*Agaricus campestris*) are the closest wild relatives of the commercially cultivated mushroom (*A. brunnescens*). They have creamy white caps, pink gills, and crisp, sweet flesh that is stronger-flavored than that of their domesticated cousins. Tim and Jane led me over a barbed-wire fence into a lush field where dairy cows grazed peacefully. It was late afternoon. The farmer, who had given us permission to enter his fields, advised us "to be careful of the bull."

In a short time we had filled our buckets. Meadow Mushrooms are not very difficult to spot, and there were so many of them in this pasture that we picked only the choicest, tightest buttons and just-opened caps, leaving the older, darker-gilled ones in the ground. There is nothing quite so tasty, I discovered, as a button-stage Meadow Mushroom, freshly plucked from the ground, neatly trimmed, wiped clean with the fingers, and popped into the mouth. I have since found that the flavor of this fungus varies and that mushrooms in one meadow may taste different from those in another.

As I was about to go after one more patch of mushrooms, the bull took exception to my presence and charged. I beat a hasty retreat to the fence and got over it very efficiently, losing only a few of the collected treats from my bucket. Bulls and barbed wire are the chief hazards of Meadow Mushroom hunting. Good exercise, fresh air, and beautiful surroundings are some of the benefits, not to mention the prospect of a delicious meal afterward.

On our way back, we stopped at the farmhouse to offer some of our collection to the farmer. "No thanks," he said, trying to conceal his horror on looking into our buckets. "I wouldn't touch those things." How convenient it is, I mused, for mycophiles to collect mushrooms on the property of mycophobes. We drove home as night was falling and prepared a wonderful repast of fresh Meadow Mushrooms sautéed in butter and sour cream, served over toast with a green salad.

Sunday morning dawned sunny and clear. Jane and I went off to a state park west of Eugene to collect Slippery Jacks. Slippery Jacks are members of a large family of mushrooms called boletes that have tubes instead of gills. Most of them are edible, although only a few are excellent; a few, those with red tube mouths, are somewhat poisonous. Slippery Jacks have beautiful canary-yellow tubes and chestnut-brown caps that are slimy when wet. We found them growing in profusion out of rich green moss at the bases of pine trees. Some were the size of a fist.

While collecting Slippery Jacks, I became aware of one of the singularities of mushroom hunting. I noticed that I could not see the mushrooms at first. Jane would run from pine tree to pine tree, exclaiming, "Oh, look! Here are more," while I would scan the ground, not seeing any until she called my attention to them. But after a short time, I began to see them, too, and before an hour was up, I was able to spot Slippery Jacks yards away. In fact, by the time we left the park with full buckets, I was so attuned to them that I would know one was at the base of a distant tree and would go right to the spot with my knife ready. On arriving, I would sometimes find nothing more than a slight crack in the moss with the tiniest patch of brown showing through. But there below, sure enough, was a choice, large button, just about to emerge in the morning sun.

Once in Colombia, while collecting San Isidro mushrooms, I had observed something similar. At first I could not find any of them, even though they were large mushrooms growing in open pastures. One of my traveling companions was very good at seeing them and to my annoyance would find mushrooms in places I had just looked. I particularly remember him coming up behind me, saying, "Hey, you just passed five." I turned around and saw a cluster of large tan mushrooms. I would swear they had not been there a moment before. I also noticed that if I walked with my friend I would see mushrooms but that if he got more than a few feet away from me, I would no longer see them. After some time and frustration, I began to see them on my own.

In Oregon, each time Jane, Tim, or another hunter would introduce me to a new species, at first I would see it only in the immediate presence of the other person and not by myself. After a period of nonseeing, the mushroom would gradually reveal itself to me. In a little while I would be able to know where a mushroom was even with minimal visual cues.

I was looking forward to cream of Slippery Jack soup

when we got home and began to clean the mushrooms. We removed the slimy peels and cut away the tubes, leaving the white flesh. Raw, it tasted sour and somewhat fruity. The acid flavor disappeared on cooking, but cream of Slippery Jack soup turned out to be disappointing. I did not care for either the texture or taste of the boletes. I later learned my gustatory intuitions were sound, because the Slippery Jacks gave me painless diarrhea. I ate them again to make sure they were the cause. They were. Slippery Jacks are now, for me, mushrooms to be admired in ways other than eating. Tim gets the same effect from them, but Jane, who likes their taste, does not, and can eat them with impunity.

My intensive course in mushrooms continued that afternoon at a spectacular mushroom show put on by the Eugene Mycological Society in the mall of a suburban shopping center. On long tables covered with beautiful fresh moss, actual specimens of most of the prominent species of the Northwest were set out for viewing, smelling, and touching. To see in the flesh all of the mushrooms I had known only from pictures was a wonderful experience. One table was heaped with Chanterelles and their close relatives, all of them delicacies. Another held the deadly amanitas. There were Shaggy Manes and Inky Caps, milky caps and coral mushrooms, puffballs and boletes. Among the boletes was a giant King Boletus (*Boletus edulis*), one of the best of the group, ranked by gourmets along with Chanterelles as one of the choicest edibles. There were mushrooms that smelled like hay and mushrooms that smelled like flour, and a blue one that smelled strongly of anise. There were mushrooms of all colors and the most fantastic shapes.

I went back to the Chanterelles and tried to fix in my mind the differences between them and similar-looking mushrooms. There is, of course, a False Chanterelle, an orange mushroom that is toxic for some persons and not for others. As I was making these observations, a young man with long hair sidled up and said to me in a low voice, "Funny, there aren't any psilocybin mushrooms here." We exchanged a few words, and it became clear that there were psilocybin mushrooms out in his car, that he would be happy to sell them to me. I had heard a great deal about psilocybin mushrooms in Oregon and was eager to learn them. A number of different active species had been reported in the region, and there was no end of secondhand information about them. But I had not yet met anyone who actually knew them.

By now I understood that one learns most mushrooms in one way only: through people who know them. It is terribly difficult to do it from books, pictures, or written descriptions, however careful. Mushroom books are notoriously unreliable and inconsistent, even to the extent of disagreeing as to whether the same species is edible or poisonous. Some of this confusion reflects a general lack of mycological study, for the world contains few qualified mycologists and their work is limited. It may also be that mushrooms vary greatly in their properties from one part of the world to another and that books written about the species of one region do not apply to those of another. In any case, books are sometimes helpful after one knows mushrooms, but they seldom help you get to know them. Until recently, the problem was compounded for psilocybin mushrooms, because so little was written about them, and what there was mostly concerned kinds that grow in Mexico.

The way to learn a mushroom, then, is to find a person who knows it and persuade that person that you are the sort who deserves to be introduced to it. Once you have met the mushroom in the field, learned to see it for yourself, and collected it, you can then introduce other worthy people to it.

My new friend at the mushroom show was named Mark. I hoped he might be a lead to the fabled psilocybin mushrooms of Oregon, but when we got to his van it turned out that what he had were small plastic bags filled with unrecognizable, frozen, chopped mushrooms. Mark was selling these for fifteen dollars a bag and said they were "very trippy" in doses of half a teaspoon. They had come from Washington State, supposedly from a commercial mushroom grower who was cultivating psilocybin mushrooms on the side. I was skeptical, but it was some sort of lead. That night Tim, Jane, and I each ate half a teaspoon of the frozen mushrooms. They tasted suspiciously like canned mushrooms. Within thirty minutes we began to feel intoxicated and eventually had strong reactions marked by stimulation, muscular incoordination, and some visual hallucinations. The effects lasted more than ten hours. Subsequent analysis of these mushrooms showed them to contain a mixture of LSD and a veterinary anesthetic called phencyclidine (PCP), a drug that causes intoxication and makes the muscles feel rubbery. PCP is a common adulterant of black-market psychedelics and often disguises the effects of LSD.* Our mushrooms, undoubtedly, were *Agaricus brunnescens*, collected from a supermarket can.

Tim, Jane, and I headed up the McKenzie River the next day into the forests of the Cascades to hunt Chanterelles. The sight of a golden-orange Chanterelle nestled in bright green moss beneath a giant Douglas Fir is about as glorious as anything could be. Chanterelles have veins on the underside instead of gills. The patterns traced by these veins are quite remarkable. A fresh Chanterelle is solid and meaty, with a pronounced aroma of apricots. The flesh is white and fibrous, looking exactly liked cooked white meat of turkey. Raw, it tastes peppery, but when slowly simmered in butter and its own juices, perhaps with a touch of sherry and herbs, it achieves culinary distinction worthy of the finest table. Enough said: You will have to try them for yourself.

---

* In recent years PCP, or "angel dust," has gained much notoriety as a new drug menace, supposed to cause mental derangement and violence. It is an unusual drug, not falling into any simple pharmacological category. It can cause hallucinations but is not a psychedelic. Some of its effects resemble those of alcohol, but it is more of a stimulant than a depressant. Many people who try it find it uninteresting; those who like it take it for the feeling of disconnection from reality it produces. Often they are young, angry people from harsh environments who have preexisting tendencies to violence. PCP is a cheap drug, easy to manufacture and widely available. I would certainly not recommend it to anyone, but neither do I consider it a "devil drug" that automatically makes people violently insane.

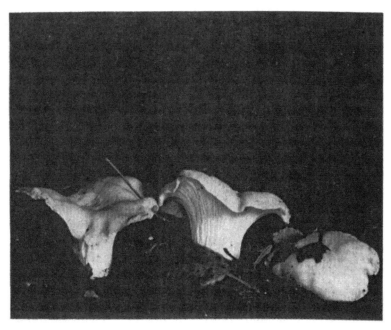

Chanterelles, *Cantharellus cibarius.* (Bob Harris)

We got twenty-five pounds of Chanterelles that day, mostly yellow ones (*Cantharellus cibarius*) but also some white ones (a closely related species, *C. subalbidus*), and some Pig's Ears (*Gomphus floccosus*), another delicious relative that is brownish on top and beautifully violet on the veined underside. We also came home with a good collection of Bloody-Juice Milky Caps (*Lactarius sanguifluus*), mushrooms that exude blood-red fluid when broken, whose flesh stains brilliant green after handling. They look like cartoon caricatures of poisonous mushrooms but are a delicious edible species that makes excellent casseroles.

*

During my stay in Oregon in the fall of 1973, I ate wild mushrooms almost every day, sometimes three times a day, usually as main courses. Perhaps because I do not eat meat, I am particularly sensitive to the meaty nature of cooked mushrooms. They resemble animal flesh more than anything vegetable, and I find them quite satisfying as the principal component of a meal. When I was eating so many wild mushrooms, I was happy, healthy, and creatively productive. Mushrooms filled my senses and thoughts and imagination. I spent many hours in the company of people who were similarly involved with mushrooms, some of them people with whom I had nothing else in common. Mycophilia cuts across all social, cultural, age, and class lines, forging real bonds of communication among otherwise disparate individuals. Mushroom consciousness is high in the Pacific Northwest, as it is also in northern California, Colorado, New England, Michigan, and Minnesota, and a few other parts of the country. Mushrooms abound in these regions, along with mushroom fanatics who hunt them down.

In view of the intensity of cravings that some of us experience for mushrooms, it is puzzling to read nutritional analyses of them, for nutritionists make mushrooms out to be very uninteresting. According to them, mushrooms contain only sixty-six calories per pound, mostly as protein, along with trace minerals and vitamins. This information leads many people to conclude that mushrooms have little worth as food and are merely useful as flavorful garnishes.

Now, the question of the food value of mushrooms really is a question about the energy content of mushrooms, for calories are a measure of available energy. Nutritionists are saying that mushrooms contain little energy relative to other foodstuffs. Yet it is clear to me that mushrooms are high in some kind of energy.

I have often eaten Shaggy Manes (*Coprinus comatus*). These delicate mushrooms and other Inky Caps are distinguished by the peculiar habit of melting into inky black liquid as they mature. Shaggy Manes come out of the ground overnight in bunches that look just like white eggs. They elongate rapidly and may be a foot above ground by midmorning. By the end of the day, there may be nothing left of them but a puddle of black liquid. This tendency to dissolve is related to their high water content, which makes them tricky to handle. They must be gathered quickly, taken home, and cooked almost immediately. Any delay or mishandling in their preparation will leave you with a puddle

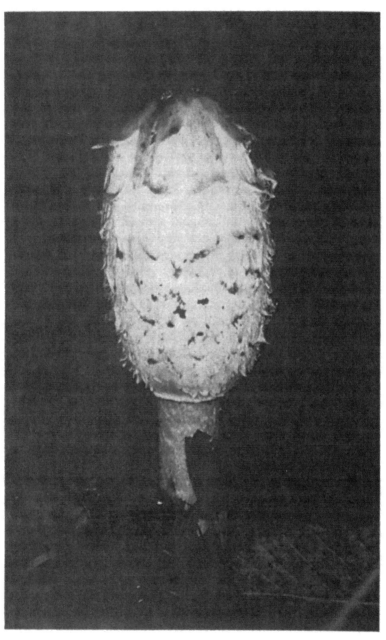

Shaggy Mane, *Coprinus comatus*. (Bob Harris)

of black liquid in your kitchen. But these fragile mushrooms come out of the ground with such relentless force that they can push up asphalt. If a driveway is laid over one of their fruiting spots, it can be broken up by the emerging mushrooms. That is evidence of energy.

Once, in suburban Washington, D.C., I found an enormous mass of brilliant orange mushrooms bursting from the stump of a dead tree on a residential street. Each cap was six inches across on a long stalk that joined many others at the base. There must have been well over a hundred in the mass. I gathered an armful, took them home, and pored over my mushroom books in hopes of making an identification. I was in luck because they were so distinctive in their appearance and habit of growth. They were the Jack-O'-Lantern Mushroom (*Omphalotus olearius* or *Clitocybe illudens*), and my book told me they should glow in the dark. I took a large cluster of them into a dark room. To my delight, the underside of each cap glowed with a brilliant blue luminescence; the light of the whole cluster was considerable. That is energy.

Mushrooms that can kill people provide further evidence of energy. Most of the deadly species are in the genus *Amanita*. They are large, beautiful mushrooms with white gills and pleasing tastes. They contain unusual chemical compounds that poison the most basic processes of cellular metabolism, leading to death through destruction of liver and kidney tissue. There is no antidote for their effects, and mortality may be over 50 percent. Symptoms do not appear until twelve to thirty-six hours after ingestion, making it impossible to remove much of the toxic material from the stomach. The devastating effects of deadly amanitas on the human organism are another clue to the nature of mushroom energy. That energy, represented in certain odd molecules, can overwhelm the balance of life.

Other mushrooms, mostly little ones in the genus *Psilocybe*, can precipitate us into the most profoundly different states of consciousness that can be utterly terrifying or inexpressibly beautiful. Anyone who has experienced their power will not dispute the statement that mushrooms are highly energetic things.

What nutritionists ought to be saying, then, is that mushrooms contain insignificant amounts of the energy nutritionists measure. That kind of energy, caloric energy, comes from the sun. Calories are simply units of solar energy bound by green plants or transformed chemically by animals that have eaten green plants. Mushrooms have little to do with the sun. Most of them are destroyed by sunlight and are best gathered in early morning before the light of day is too intense. Human societies in all parts of the world associate mushrooms with the moon. This association may not be fanciful. Friends of mine who lived near the village of Silvia in the Colombian state of Cauca told me that the growth of San Isidro mushrooms there was correlated with phases of the moon: Whenever rainfall was sufficient, a new crop would appear each time the moon waxed, disappearing just after the full.

Many people also associate mushrooms with water, the feminine or lunar element, as opposed to fire, which is masculine and solar. Not only do mushrooms contain high percentages of water, their growth is triggered primarily by rain. When I have picked mushrooms in wet forests on misty mornings after fall rains, they have seemed to me to be entirely creations of water.

Some years ago, before I had met many wild mushrooms, I came across a line in a macrobiotic cookbook that made no sense to me: "Mushrooms are about as *yin* as you can comfortably get." The book warned against eating many of them. I was familiar with the Chinese-Taoist concept of *yin* and *yang* as the fundamental dualism in the universe, but I could not picture any scale of foodstuffs on which mushrooms were so far toward one end that they were dangerous to eat.

More recently, I met a young woman in Marin County, California, who told me she had been poisoned seriously by the Panther Amanita (*A. pantherina*). Panther Amanitas look like Fly Amanitas, but the color of the cap is tan instead of red. I asked her for details of her experience. She said she

had been living with a man in the far north of California
with little money and little food. One day two "beautiful
brown mushrooms the size of baseballs" came up on their
lawn. Knowing nothing about mushrooms, they decided
these were a "gift from heaven." She picked them, sliced
them, and fried them with onions. They tasted good. Thirty
minutes after eating the dish, she felt "sicker than I ever felt
in my life — not just in my stomach but all through my
body." She next experienced a "vivid awareness of my life
processes shutting down from the outside in" until all that
was left was a tiny flame of consciousness. Then that flick-
ered out. She regained awareness in a hospital. She and her
friend had been found unconscious and been taken for medical help. Their stomachs were pumped, and with supportive
therapy, they were ready for discharge twenty-four hours
later. "I couldn't look at a mushroom again for six months,"
she concluded.

As this woman recounted her adventure, I had a sudden
flash of illumination about the warning in the macrobiotic
cookbook. For one of the classic descriptions of the yin force
is "contraction toward a center," as opposed to "expansion
from a center," which is yang. The Panther Amanita had
overwhelmed her organism with a heavy dose of yin energy,
the dark lunar force that kills by inward reduction to a di-
mensionless point. That is death by water. Panther Amanitas, producing symptoms rapidly, seldom if ever kill, although they can be very toxic. The truly deadly amanitas, like
the Death Cup, do not cause noticeable effects until their yin
energy is disseminated through the body.

Mushrooms are primal symbols of the lunar force. I do not
mean simply that they represent it but that they actually
embody it, and here, I think, is the real basis for the fear of
mushrooms that crops up again and again among human beings. A Mexican term for mushrooms is *carne de los muertos*,
"flesh of the dead." In fact, cemeteries are good collecting
grounds for mushrooms. Besides bringing death, the lunar
force can cause madness (lunacy), and in the case of psilocybin mushrooms, the symbolism holds true.

Now, it is clear that many persons regard manifestations

of lunar energy as evil. Death and madness are commonly considered evils that afflict mankind. Night, the full moon, and female witchcraft are a sinister trio. But it should be obvious that the dark side of existence is integrally part of things. Night and day make up one cycle of existence. Life without death is unthinkable. The moon and sun in the sky are outward expressions of the complementary interaction of the opposite forces of the universe.

In human experience, lunar forces manifest themselves in the life of the unconscious: in dreams, intuitions, trances, and all states of consciousness where what is normally hidden from awareness breaks through. We cannot possibly do away with those forces in the outside world because we carry them around within us. It is even possible that external manifestations of those forces, such as mushrooms, are projections or creations of our internal energies. Because our mental life is usually dominated by masculine, solar forces, we tend to think of our dark sides as nonexistent or evil. Chinese philosophy is very clear on the wrongness of that way of thinking. *I Ching* or *Book of Changes*, which describes the interplay of yin and yang in the world, says of the yin force: "In itself, of course, the Receptive [yin] is just as important as the Creative [yang], but the attribute of devotion defines the place occupied by this primal power in relation to the Creative. For the Receptive must be activated and led by the Creative; then it is productive of good. Only when it abandons this position and tries to stand as an equal side by side with the Creative, does it become evil."*

Nutritionists do not see the reality of the lunar energy of mushrooms; measuring the traces of solar energy in them, they conclude that mushrooms are not very nourishing. Macrobiotic faddists come close to regarding mushrooms as dangerous. In yoga dietetics, mushrooms are assigned to the lowest of three energy groups of foods: the *tamasic*, a category that also includes spoiled and rotten things and other

* Cary F. Baynes and Richard Wilhelm, trans., *I Ching, or Book of Changes*, 3rd ed., Bollingen Series, no. 19 (Princeton, N.J.: Princeton University Press, 1967), p. 11.

items to be avoided by yogis. Are mushrooms genuinely harmful to aspirants on spiritual paths? Or is it that followers of yoga, a male-dominated system, are uneasy about their own lunar natures and project that concern onto mushrooms?

The energy of mushrooms is real and strong: Remember, it can push up asphalt, unhinge the mind, kill, and permeate the darkness with eerie, heatless light. Where does that energy go when it enters the body? What does it nourish other than the physical body that requires calories?

I do not think it unreasonable that lunar energy is food for the unconscious, that mushrooms in the diet stimulate the imagination and intuition. Wild mushrooms are stronger in this respect than cultivated ones, and this line of speculation explains to me the passionate enthusiasm of mushroomers. I am not suggesting that mushrooms are required for the health of the unconscious or that they are the only means of stimulating the activity of that sphere. But they are a means, and those who feel attracted to them should follow their call.

I have written that no line exists between psychedelic and poisonous varieties. From one point of view, mushrooms are simply mushrooms, all of them expressions and embodiments of the basic energy represented by the moon. I doubt that canned mushrooms deliver much of that energy to the mind, but fresh cultivated ones certainly give us some. Chanterelles, Shaggy Manes, morels, and other choice wild fungi are higher in lunar nutritive factors. Psilocybin mushrooms are so rich in them that they can open our normal waking consciousness to experiences that usually remain below awareness. Some amanitas — the Panther and the Fly — are so strong that they can make us sick. Yet some people use them deliberately to change consciousness. Other amanitas are too powerful for our beings; they flood the system with fatal doses of yin.

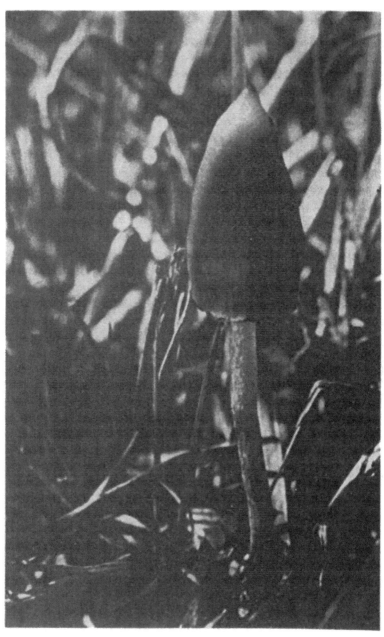

The Liberty Cap, *Psilocybe semilanceata*. (Bob Harris)

9

MUSHROOMS III

ALTHOUGH I SATISFIED all of my cravings for wild
mushrooms in 1973 and made friends with a great many
varieties, I did poorly at tracking down the psilocybin
mushrooms of Oregon. By the end of October I had resigned
myself to not finding them. Since I was feeling the urge to
migrate southward, I packed up my things and made ready
to leave for Arizona. On my way out of Eugene I was stopped
by a man who introduced himself as Richard, a friend of a
friend. He said he knew people on the Oregon coast who
were collecting and using psilocybin mushrooms. If I could
stay another day, he would drive me to them.

So, on Hallowe'en, in the midst of heavy downpour, four
of us drove over the coastal mountains to the gray Pacific,
where we met Greg and Susan. They told us they knew a
psychoactive mushroom called the Liberty Cap that grew in
cow pastures near the coast and said they would take us to
them. The six of us drove north through the storm, along the
coast into Lincoln County, where we turned inland through
rich meadows. Susan told us the Liberty Caps had been
growing in abundance all month.

We stopped by a large field that looked partly flooded. It
was cold and raw and wet. Greg and Susan got into their
rain gear. I had not yet learned how to dress like a proper
Oregonian and was soaked through within minutes of our
descent from the road to the inevitable barbed-wire fence. It
was hard to believe that mushrooms would be growing in
such inclement conditions.

We fanned out through the sodden field with instructions to show any likely mushrooms to Susan or Greg. In some places the grass was under several inches of cold rainwater.

"Here they are," Susan finally called out. She indicated several little mushrooms growing in a small group. At first glance they were quite uninteresting. Their color was dingy gray-brown, and they were barely distinguishable from the tall grass in which they grew.

Close up, the Liberty Caps were more distinctive. I had never seen caps of that particular shape: conical, with a pronounced point or nipple at the top. The flesh of the cap was so thin that it was translucent, especially near the margin; the wet, outer surface was glistening and slimy. There were clear vertical striations around the margin. The stipe (stem) had an elastic pliancy that allowed the mushroom to be flopped back and forth without breaking it. The caps were about one centimeter in diameter at the broadest point, on seven-centimeter stipes. I found it incredible that such tiny, delicate mushrooms could be so powerful. The psilocybin mushroom I knew from Latin America was robust and fleshy.

"How many of them do you eat?" I asked.

"I like to eat twenty," Greg said. "I've eaten up to a hundred."

"What is that like?"

"Well, you lie on the ground unable to move for a couple of hours. It's O.K. But twenty is a good solid dose."

"Sometimes, I'll just eat two or three on a really nice day, in the morning," Susan said. "I like to trip on them, too, but just a few in the morning make you feel really alive. All the colors of everything stand out, and your body feels energized."

Soon, other people began to find Liberty Caps, although, as usual, I had trouble seeing them for some time and could only notice them if I was walking near Greg or Susan.

The collection thus far was divided up, and we each got about six Liberty Caps. I chewed on mine slowly, savoring their strongly wild mushroom flavor. Then I set about gathering more. Before long I began to notice Liberty Caps — one here, one there. I ate them as I found them. Soon I had eaten twenty-five of the tiny mushrooms. I was soaked to the skin but excited enough not to mind. As I found new mushrooms, I put them into a plastic container.

Gradually I became aware of a strange sensation in my stomach, a sort of buzzing vibration that grew slowly in intensity. It was not unpleasant, and I knew at once it was the mushrooms. Over the next ten minutes this unusual feeling became stronger, filling my abdomen. Then it began to invade the rest of my body, pushing outward through the muscles to the extremities. I was distinctly aware of a subtle but powerful energy vibrating through the musculature of my whole body. It made me feel warm and strong. As it reached my head, my senses sharpened, and I found myself admiring qualities of the wet pasture I had ignored until then. The green of the grass was of glowing intensity, highlighted by tones of brown and red. The smell of the earth and rain was overpowering. I had no desire to move. If the ground had been dry, I would have stretched out and rolled in the grass.

Our little group slowly drew together. Obviously, we were all feeling the effects of the mushrooms. We moved slowly and gracefully, swinging our arms and laughing at each other. The laughter seemed to bubble up from inside, and the sound of it echoed inside my chest. I was also very conscious of the taste of the mushrooms. It was as strong as if fresh in my mouth but was diffused through my whole body. I felt the taste in my muscles.

The rain picked up in intensity. Clearly, we could not stay out in the field much longer. It was late afternoon and turning colder. Slowly we wended our way out of the pasture, across the fence, and up a steep bank to the car. I curled up in a corner of the back seat as we started to move. It was an hour's drive south along the coast to Greg and Susan's house.

The mushroom energy continued to course around my body. Now it began to pull me away from ordinary awareness into a realm that bordered on sleep but was not sleep. It was an effort to maintain awareness of the car and my fellow passengers, let alone the scenery outside. Instead, I closed my eyes and began to see visions that were somewhere between images in the mind's eye and actual movies projected on the insides of my eyelids. At first there were shadowy patterns that tended to multiply themselves in infinite regressions, but these soon resolved themselves into very clear images of mushrooms. The mushrooms that appeared to me were of one type, not Liberty Caps. They grew in clustered bunches, the stipes arising from a common point, and lacked the Liberty Cap's distinctive peak. They were also fleshier and bigger. I had never seen them before. Bunches of these visionary mushrooms appeared out of nowhere, springing up at odd angles, swirling, and receding. They occupied my attention completely until we arrived back at the house.

It was now a stormy Hallowe'en night, and a long ride home through the mountains lay between us and Eugene. The visions were subsiding, and I volunteered to drive. It took some concentration to follow the tortuous road through the rain, but we arrived home without incident. I could still feel the vibrational energy in my muscles, though it was fading rapidly. About six hours after I ate the mushrooms, I was back to normal, feeling tired. I fell asleep quickly and awoke the next morning refreshed.

In the following months, I made an effort to find out more about Liberty Caps and eventually met an Oregon State University student of mycology, who told me the mushroom appeared to be a species called *Psilocybe semilanceata*. Like all psilocybes it has purplish-brown spores, and like all psychoactive psilocybes, it tends to stain blue on handling or drying. Liberty Caps appear only after the autumn equinox and continue to grow until the winter solstice or beyond, despite low temperatures. Their range extends from the California border north into British Columbia, from the ocean east to the crest of the coastal mountains. The mushrooms grow in actively used cow pastures. It is likely that cows eat them in the course of their grazing and help propagate them by spreading the spores in their manure. Whether cows experience any effects from them is a moot question.

Collecting Liberty Caps is not all that easy. In many fields the mushrooms are sparse, and they hide themselves well in the midst of clumps of tall grass. Sometimes you have to crawl on your hands and knees to spot them, pulling apart the tufts of grass. Then there is the usual problem of not being able to see them at first. I am convinced that the ability to see mushrooms is independent of visual acuity. It has more to do with pattern recognition, something that goes on in the higher brain. One can stare at a mushroom, even a large one, and not recognize it. Sometimes I almost think the mushrooms themselves decide when and to whom to reveal their presence.

I discovered that knowledge of Liberty Caps was not widespread in inland communities in Oregon in the early 1970s but that many coastal residents knew how to collect them. A few users told me they were called Liberty Caps because they resembled the Liberty Bell in Philadelphia, a resemblance I could not see. I discarded that theory when I received a letter from a friend in Wales telling me that people in that country were getting high on mushrooms called Liberty Caps or Pixie Caps. The letter contained some dried specimens; it was the same mushroom.

Given the fact that inhabitants of the British Isles call this little mushroom the Liberty Cap, it is certain that the name comes from the French cap of liberty, a symbol of the French Revolution that appears on coins of the period. That symbol, in turn, derives from the Phrygian bonnet of Roman times, given to slaves upon emancipation. The Oxford English Dictionary describes the Phrygian bonnet as "a conical cap with the peak bent or turned over in the front, worn by the ancient Phrygians and in modern times identified with the 'cap of liberty.'" Especially on drying, *Psilocybe semilanceata* takes on the appearance of this ancient symbol.

I learned how to dry Liberty Caps by spreading them on a screen where there is good air circulation. In less than twenty-four hours, they are crisp and dry, their caps crinkly

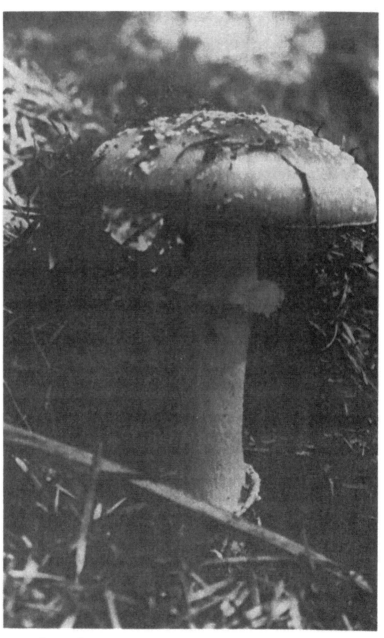

The Panther Amanita, *Amanita pantherina*. (Jeremy Bigwood)

with a metallic sheen, sometimes showing streaks of blue. In this state they keep their potency for a year or more. In my experiments with these mushrooms, I found I preferred them dried to fresh and suspect that some mildly toxic constituents disappear on drying. It is convenient to make a tea of them by steeping the ground, dried material in freshly boiled water. Liberty Caps are more powerful when taken on an empty stomach. I found them better at night if I wished to concentrate on the visions seen with the eyes closed. They have a great potential to stimulate the visual imagination and open people to unconscious forces.

I do not wish to minimize the negative aspects of Liberty Caps. Because they deliver a strong dose of lunar energy, they are quite capable of plunging people into dark and terrifying spaces, of showing us the hollow madness and sickness of ourselves and the world. No one should risk this experience who is not prepared to confront it. The use of psilocybin mushrooms as casual, recreational intoxicants is risky in this way. Natural psychedelics as strong as Liberty Caps should be reserved for special occasions and used deliberately with adequate preparation.

I have searched through standard mushroom books to find references to *Psilocybe semilanceata* but have found it only in one European handbook, which called it a poisonous species. No doubt, persons who ate it unawares, without the proper mind set, could interpret the dramatic changes as mushroom poisoning.

Really, there are no differences between drugs and poisons except in dosage. All drugs in high enough doses are poisons, and many poisons at low enough doses cause interesting and useful drug effects. Except in very toxic dose ranges, expectation or set may play the critical role in determining whether a person is poisoned by a psychoactive drug or taken on a pleasant trip. The most dramatic example of the power of expectation I have ever come across concerns another mushroom of the Pacific Northwest, the Panther Amanita, *Amanita pantherina*.

Mycologists say that this large brown *Amanita* is the most

common cause of serious mushroom poisoning in the western United States. It is not deadly, like some of its relatives, but it certainly can make people quite sick. Nevertheless, it has become a popular recreational drug in Oregon and Washington, much to the bafflement of mycologists. Until recently, books wrongly identified the active agent of *A. pantherina* as muscarine, an alkaloid known from other mushrooms that stimulates the parasympathetic nervous system, causing such symptoms as profuse sweating and salivation. In this wrong belief, the books also recommended treating intoxication by the Panther Amanita with injections of atropine, a well-known drug from the nightshade family of higher plants that counteracts the effects of muscarine. In fact, we know now that the real active agent of *A. pantherina* is muscimol, a drug whose effects are potentiated by atropine.

I was interested in tracking down cases of ingestion of the panther amanita in the Pacific Northwest and soon found that they were of two kinds.* Some people ate the mushroom by accident. They were foraging for edible species and made a mistake. Thinking the Panther was some innocuous edible, they took it home, cooked it, and ate it. This mushroom produces an intoxication of rapid onset. Within fifteen to thirty minutes it made all of these people feel very peculiar.

Now, none of them had had any contact with the drug subculture. Their only prior experience with psychoactive substances had been with alcohol, tobacco, and coffee. Also, like many mushroom hunters in the English-speaking world, these people were unconsciously mycophobic. When they began to feel peculiar, all of them decided they had eaten a poisonous species and were about to die. One woman first called her lawyer to change an item in her will, then summoned an ambulance. All of them got sick. All lost con-

---

* Some of these cases were first described by Jonathan Ott in his article, "Psycho-Mycological Studies of *Amanita:* From Ancient Sacrament to Modern Phobia," *Journal of Psychedelic Drugs* 8, no. 1 (1976): 27–35.

sciousness for varying periods of time, from a few minutes to a half-hour. All were taken to emergency wards of hospitals, where they uniformly received incorrect medical treatment: large doses of atropine that made their conditions worse. They were admitted to medical wards and discharged in thirty-six to forty-eight hours, since it is the nature of this intoxication to subside quickly, usually within twelve hours. Most of these victims said they would never hunt mushrooms again. One man said he could not look at mushrooms in the store for months afterward. When told that some people ate the same mushroom for fun, they shook their heads in disbelief.

The other cases of Panther Amanita ingestion I uncovered occurred in members of the drug subculture who ate the mushroom deliberately because they heard it gave a high. These people had extensive experience with marijuana and hallucinogens, including psilocybin mushrooms. They believed that nature provides us with all sorts of natural highs just waiting to be picked in the woods. When these people felt the rapid effects of *Amanita pantherina*, they welcomed them as signs that the mushroom was really working. None of them got sick. (A few mentioned transient nausea but did not regard it as important.) None of them lost consciousness. None of them felt it necessary to summon help. All of them liked the experience and most said they intended to repeat it. Some had already eaten the Panther a number of times.

When I present this information to groups of physicians, they try hard to come up with some simple, materialistic explanation for the difference in response of the two kinds of cases. A question they always ask is: "Might there have been a dose difference?" The answer is, yes, there was a dose difference; the people who ate the Panther deliberately ate more of it than the people who ate it accidentally.

The only way to interpret this story is by reference to set. The Panther mushroom produces a powerful but neutral change in psychophysiology. People with strong fears can turn this feeling into mushroom poisoning by concentrating on its negative aspects and, eventually, by putting themselves in the hands of others who actually do make them feel worse. People with strong hopes of a new high can turn the same feeling into a welcome state by ignoring the negative aspects and concentrating on the interesting changes in mood and perception. Although Liberty Caps are much less toxic than Panther Amanitas, I have no doubt that the same kinds of differences would show up between people who eat them unawares and people who eat them deliberately.

*

During the spring and summer months, when no Liberty Caps are available, Oregonians can use another variety of psilocybin mushroom in the genus *Panaeolus*. It is easily collected in quantity on piles of rotting hay in manured cow fields in the Willamette Valley, where most of the population of the state lives. This mushroom, *Panaeolus subbalteatus*, though small, is twice as fleshy as the Liberty Cap. Yet the dose is the same: twenty mushrooms. That is to say, the *Panaeolus* is less potent. Moreover, the quality of the effect is not as good. Particularly when fresh, it tends to produce symptoms of mild toxicity. Some people experience nausea from it. I get an uncomfortable restlessness for an hour after eating it. This toxicity is reduced on drying, but not eliminated. *Panaeolus subbalteatus* is less effective at triggering visual spectacles. Nonetheless, it is a popular mushroom during the warm months.

As many as a dozen other active species grow in the Pacific Northwest. Some of these are woodland species that are weaker than the Liberty Cap. Collecting little brown mushrooms in woods is much riskier than doing the same thing in open pastures. Several species of the genus *Galerina* that grow on wood or buried wood contain the same toxins as the deadly amanitas and can kill, and sometimes they grow very near psilocybes of the same size. No one should look for psilocybin mushrooms under shrubs and trees who has not learned to recognize galerinas.

Many collectors of Liberty Caps and *Panaeolus subbal-*

teatus have little knowledge of mushrooms in general. I have met many hunters of these magic mushrooms who do not know how to collect Meadow Mushrooms or Chanterelles. Yet I have heard of no cases of poisonings of people looking for psilocybin mushrooms in open cow fields, at least not in the Northwest. In the Gulf South, where the principal species is *Psilocybe cubensis*, the large San Isidro mushroom, I have met people who got sick to their stomachs by eating the wrong kinds, but I still have uncovered no cases of anything worse.

One of the more powerful woodland species of *Psilocybe* is *P. baeocystis*, which occurs throughout western Oregon and Washington. It is a larger mushroom than the Liberty Cap, and two caps may be sufficient for a strong experience. In the fall of 1974, *P. baeocystis* turned up in large numbers on the mulch under rhododendron bushes in a municipal park in the middle of Eugene. Many people collected and used it.

Psilocybe cyanescens is another woodland psilocybin mushroom that grows abundantly in Oregon and Washington and is much prized by collectors. It grows on bark mulches in large, bunched clusters, and is more potent than most of its relatives, one to four of the small mushrooms being a good dose. *P. cyanescens* is a beautiful fungus with wavy cap margins that turn blue quite readily. Blue Halos and Wavy Caps are two common names I have heard for it. Unlike the other species of the Pacific Northwest, this one lends itself easily to cultivation.

Still other species keep turning up. A new member of *Psilocybe* began growing heavily on the campus of the University of Washington in Seattle in the fall of 1973. Word of it got out quickly, and students began eating it, to the consternation of university officials. The mushroom appeared to be spreading by way of a bark mulch used by the buildings and grounds crew — at least, each time a new area of the campus was mulched, it came up in great numbers. This mushroom has since been named *Psilocybe stuntzii* in honor of Dr. Daniel Stuntz, professor emeritus of mycology at the University of Washington.

During a trip to Washington State in October 1974, I found this mushroom on a lawn in front of a commercial nursery just south of the state capital at Olympia. It was first discovered there by an Oregon collector now living near Olympia, who noticed the mushroom on the lawn, tried it, and confirmed its activity. *P. stuntzii* is a lovely, chestnut-brown, fleshy mushroom that turns blue readily and has a persistent annulus, or veil, around the upper stipe, an unusual character in this genus. Some users call it the Washington Blue Veil and consider it very desirable, although it is somewhat less potent than the Liberty Cap. It grows in clusters, the stipes arising from a common point. When I first met them in Olympia, I recognized them at once as the mushrooms I had seen in the visions of my first Liberty Cap experience.

I chatted with the owner of the nursery about his lawn. He had not failed to notice large numbers of young people, especially students from nearby Evergreen State College, crawling about on his property picking mushrooms. "Sometimes it gets so bad, I have to turn on the sprinklers to get rid of them," he complained. I explained to him what the mushrooms were, assured him that no one was likely to get hurt by them, and got permission to collect specimens for identification. He told me his staff had prepared hundreds of similar lawns throughout Olympia using the same mulch and manure. *P. stuntzii* will probably turn up all over the state capital.

I hear of people picking psilocybin mushrooms in New York State, Maine, Indiana, Tennessee, California, and in eastern and western Canada. It looks as if they are nearly everywhere and that people who go out knowing what to look for will find them. I see no way that any government agency can control the spread of these mushrooms or of the knowledge of their properties. They are with us to stay and doubtless will be more and more in evidence.

Have they always been here and not been noticed until recently? Or are they appearing in new locations? The story of *P. stuntzii* at the University of Washington suggests that

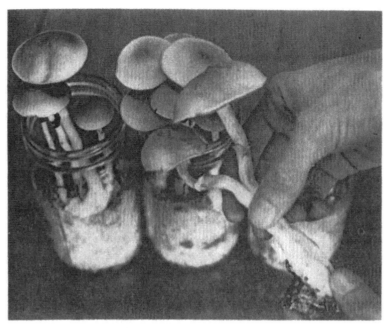

Psilocybe cubensis in cultivation on a medium of grain. (Jeremy Bigwood)

psilocybin mushrooms are really on the march. Certainly, human involvement with them is now a factor helping to disseminate them.

In recent years, an explosion of psychoactive mushroom use has occurred in the Pacific Northwest and elsewhere. Four conferences on hallucinogenic mushrooms took place between 1976 and 1979.

In the fall of 1975, extremely heavy fruitings of the Liberty Cap in Oregon permitted collectors to gather enough mushrooms to sell them. In Eugene, Liberty Caps sold for $75 to $100 a pound, wet weight. One consequence of all the collecting was a great deal of publicity in the newspapers, along with many complaints from farmers about trespassers. Public anxiety about hallucinogenic mushrooms increased in Oregon over the next few years, and police began arresting pickers for trespassing.

Some farmers attempted to cope with the problem by charging admission to their fields. A few even provided pickers with pails for a fee and charged by the hour. In 1978 the Oregon legislature passed a law making it illegal to possess the mushrooms or allow them to grow on your property — clearly an unenforceable law.

A development with wider implications is the perfection of simple techniques for home cultivation of psilocybin mushrooms. A number of companies now sell by mail kits to grow the mushrooms and spores of the common species. Federal law controls all "materials" containing psilocybin. Spores of the mushrooms do not contain the drug and are legal, although they produce illegal material when they germinate. Growing mushrooms from spores is not as easy as growing higher plants from seeds, but many people have learned to do it, especially with *Psilocybe cubensis*. As a result, that mushroom is now available all over America.

Meanwhile, general mushroom consciousness continues to mushroom. Mycological societies report rapid growth of membership. Sales of mushroom books keep rising. Consumer demand for fresh mushrooms keeps growing, and a few exotic species are now obtainable in some markets, including fresh Oyster Mushrooms and fresh Chinese black mushrooms.

The essence of the revolution in consciousness occurring all about us is the emergence of unconscious forces long denied by our culture and the beginnings of attempts to integrate them into the fabric of our individual and social lives. Mushrooms are external symbols of those forces, and their invasion of our outward lives is a dramatic and encouraging sign of the progress of this change.

10

MARIJUANA RECONSIDERED

MARIJUANA IS STILL the subject of such heated debate that it is hard to get useful answers to simple questions like, "Is it healthy to use marijuana?" or "What are its medicinal properties?" I have studied this controversial plant for a long time and have come to some definite conclusions about it.

Cannabis is one of the oldest known useful plants. It is so closely allied with human beings that we cannot unravel its ancestral history. Truly wild hemp, completely independent of man, is unknown. Cannabis provides us with an edible seed, an edible oil, a fiber, a medicine, and a psychoactive drug. That is a lot for one plant to do, which is why it has always been an important cultivated crop.

In our society, most people who use cannabis smoke it for its psychoactive effect: They use it to get high. I am a great believer in the value of being high. High states of consciousness show us the potentials of our nervous systems. They help us integrate mind and body. They promote health. And they feel good. There are many ways to get high. You can do it through music, dance, athletics, sex, fasting, meditation, drugs, and countless other techniques.

That so many different methods lead to the same experiences suggests that the experiences come from inside us, that they are latent in the human nervous system, waiting to be released. It is important to keep this idea in mind in considering drugs. Drugs do not contain highs; they do not put any experiences into us that are not there already. They sim-

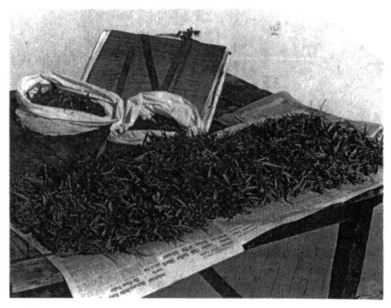

Freshly harvested flowering tops of marijuana. This is a resin-rich variety from India. (S. K. Sharma)

ply make us feel physically different for a time, and if we are set to interpret that change in a certain way, we can use it as an opportunity to let ourselves feel high.

Marijuana, by its direct pharmacological actions, causes a number of subtle changes in our mind-body. For example, it increases heart rate, dries up saliva and tears, and alters body perception. These changes are so slight that novice users may not notice them at all. Some people may feel them but not associate them with any interesting changes in consciousness. On the other hand, regular users of marijuana come to associate the changed feeling with a high. That is to say, being high on marijuana is a learned association between an experience that is always on tap within the nervous system and a change in feeling caused by the drug.

Most people who ask questions about marijuana want to know whether it is good or bad. (Usually, they have already decided.) But drugs in themselves are neither good nor bad. They are just drugs, with potentials for both constructive

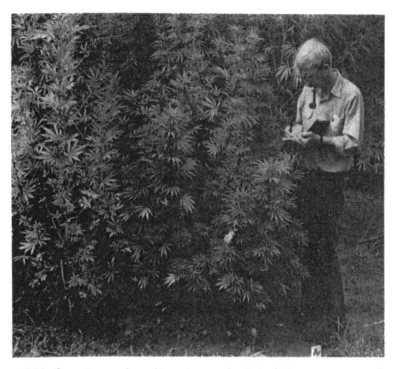

A field of marijuana, *Cannabis sativa*, at the United States government's experimental farm in Mississippi. (Timothy Plowman)

and destructive uses. One reason that research on marijuana is mostly unenlightening is that many researchers set out to prove the goodness or badness of the substance without realizing that they are imposing their own values on it. There has been an enormous amount of research on cannabis in the past ten years. One investigator has commented that we now know more about marijuana than we do about penicillin. Most of this information is irrelevant to our concerns about the drug and gives us little help in deciding what to do with it. A great deal of it is contradictory, reflecting the differing biases of researchers.

Although I feel marijuana is neither good nor bad of itself, I have no hesitation in talking about good or bad uses people make of it. We cannot discuss psychoactive drugs meaningfully apart from people, for everything interesting about the drugs arises from the relationships people form with them.

What are the characteristics of a good relationship with marijuana? A primary aspect of a good relationship with any psychoactive drug is awareness of its nature. When people forget that drugs are drugs, they are on the road to trouble. Look at the extent of serious dependence on coffee in our society. Coffee is a strong psychoactive drug; its direct pharmacological effects are more powerful than those of cannabis. Dependence on it has a marked physiological component. Many coffee-dependent persons suffer withdrawal syndromes each morning: They are incoordinated, unable to think clearly, and unable to move their bowels until they have their first fix of coffee. Yet most of these people are unaware that they are in a bad relationship with a drug, let alone a strong drug. To them coffee is just a beverage they like to drink.

Another characteristic of a good relationship with a drug is getting a positive and useful effect from it. In the case of marijuana that means getting high when you smoke it. The first thing that goes wrong in relationships with drugs when we use them too frequently is that the experiences we seek in them diminish in intensity. If we keep on using the drugs more and more frequently, the highs will disappear altogether, and we will find ourselves using them just to relieve negative symptoms.

The explanation of this pattern is that highs are not direct effects of drugs but indirect associations between the feelings drugs cause and experiences waiting to be released in our nervous systems. When we use any drug very frequently, the novelty of the feelings it causes wears off. It no longer makes us feel as different as it did initially and so does not serve as well as a trigger for a high. That is why many people report the first highs they ever had from any drug to be the best and why people who are heavily dependent on drugs do not get very intense experiences from them.

Frequency of use is the critical factor. But it is not possible to say what is too frequent use except with reference to a specific individual. For one person, smoking marijuana twice a week may be too much, but for another, smoking four times a day may not be too much. The only criterion is whether the person is able to maintain highs at a given level of use. If you are using marijuana regularly and find that you do not get as high from it as you used to, that is a warning that you are using it too much.

Ironically, many people who begin to lose the high of marijuana as a result of too frequent use try to get it back by smoking more or looking for stronger pot. Of course, those actions simply make the problem worse. Stronger pot may work for a while, but soon you will be in the same predicament as before. The only solution is to abstain from use for a while and then resume at a lower frequency. In general, any psychoactive drug is most effective when used least frequently. Furthermore, people who ignore or misunderstand the significance of highs that diminish with increasing frequency of use will eventually find that they cannot easily stop using the drug.

A third characteristic of a good relationship with a drug like marijuana is ease of separation from it. Can you take it or leave it? Do you always smoke a joint if it is offered to you? How long have you gone without the drug since becoming a user? These are hard questions, especially since we often play games with ourselves about our habits. (Remember Mark Twain's comment about quitting cigarettes: "To cease smoking is the easiest thing I ever did; I ought to know because I've done it a thousand times.") Dependence on marijuana is subtle and not marked by prominent physiological changes like dependence on coffee or alcohol. But heavy marijuana smoking can be a neurotic habit, both unproductive and difficult to break.

As a marijuana user, then, if you remain aware that you are using a drug, if you are able to maintain your highs over time, if you can separate yourself from the use of marijuana easily, and if you do not experience any adverse effects on your health, then you have a good relationship with that substance.

The opposite characteristics mark bad relationships with marijuana. I meet many heavy users who do not consider marijuana a drug. It is just a "smoking herb" to them. Some of these users smoke marijuana day in and day out and do not get as high on it as they did when they first began smoking. They are always on the lookout for stronger forms, such as Thai sticks, potent Hawaiian, or preparations of hash oil. They cannot separate themselves from this habitual use of marijuana and are very good at rationalizing it. ("Oh, John just came in; let's roll another joint." "We can't eat that ice cream without smoking some Hawaiian." "We've got to get really stoned before we go to the movie.") Some of these people suffer adverse consequences of marijuana on health, although they often deny them.

The final characteristic of a good relationship with any psychoactive drug is that no impairment of health occurs, even over time. The greatest health hazard of marijuana seems to me to be its irritating effect on the respiratory tract. It is unfortunate that smoking has become the universal mode of consuming cannabis in our part of the world. Hemp drugs can be eaten, of course. They are more powerful by mouth, take longer to come on, and produce different effects. It is healthier to eat marijuana than to smoke it, but it is also more trouble to prepare, and few smokers like to eat it except on occasion.

I meet many marijuana smokers with chronic, dry coughs, typical of bronchial irritation. Many of these people are unaware of their coughing and resentful of having it pointed out to them. One of the silliest scenes of New Age life that I have witnessed again and again is a roomful of people coughing their heads off over some especially harsh preparation of cannabis and pronouncing it "really good stuff."

As we have all read, scientists have attributed a great many horrible medical effects to marijuana, from brain damage to chromosomal damage, but in most cases the research is shoddy, using poor controls and demonstrating mainly the researchers' own prejudices. A few findings are worth mentioning.

Several investigators have reported that marijuana impairs the immune system in human beings by interfering with the activity of certain white blood cells. The workers who first described this effect were rabid antimarijuana crusaders, but some less biased investigators have supported their findings. Other experiments contradict them. Most of the evidence comes from test-tube studies rather than clinical research in real people. Epidemiological studies in populations that use marijuana heavily give us no reason to believe that users are more prone to infections than nonusers. Therefore, the test-tube results, even if confirmed, may have no clinical significance.

Another research finding, much publicized in the past few years, is that marijuana use may decrease blood levels of the male hormone testosterone in men. Again, there are contradictory experiments, and the issue is not settled. Of course, even if marijuana does have this effect, its significance is not clear. High testosterone levels may correlate more with aggressiveness than with sexual adjustment; some men in our society might benefit from a reduction in this hormone.

A more bizarre effect, also well publicized, is that marijuana may stimulate the development of breasts in some men. At first glance, this looks like fantastic antimarijuana propaganda, but, in fact, there are a few documented cases of male users who have developed breasts. This condition, called gynecomastia, is normally quite rare. The active compounds of marijuana have some molecular resemblance to certain female hormones (estrogens). Possibly, some men are born with a biochemical idiosyncrasy that causes their bodies to mistake the chemicals in hemp for estrogens. This susceptibility is uncommon, and only a tiny percentage of male users is at risk.

In general, marijuana is a relatively nontoxic drug, especially in comparison with other psychoactive drugs in common use, such as alcohol, tobacco, coffee, and tranquilizers. I repeat that the greatest hazard to health seems to be the irritation from smoking, and individuals are more or less likely to develop respiratory conditions as a result of this irritation. If you are prone to chest colds and bronchitis, be careful.

So far I have talked about the use of cannabis as a psychoactive drug. What about its use as a remedy? The plant has a long and distinguished history of use in medicine

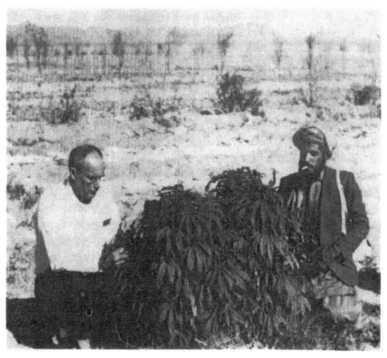

Cannabis indica in Afghanistan. This dwarf form of marijuana has broad leaflets and a very high resin content. It is the source of hashish and of the medicinal preparations of cannabis used formerly in Western medicine. (R. E. Schultes)

around the world. It was extremely popular in Europe and America in the nineteenth century in the form of a tincture and was used for all sorts of conditions.

The attractiveness of cannabis as a medicine is that it is both powerful and nontoxic. Its ability to make people feel different, especially when they consume it orally, puts it in quite another class from herbs like peppermint and chamomile. Its safety, even in large overdoses, makes it much easier to use than drugs like opium and belladonna.

In nineteenth-century medicine, tincture of cannabis was used mainly as a sedative and antispasmodic. It was dispensed for insomnia, migraine, epilepsy, excitability, childbirth, and menstrual discomfort. Interestingly enough, the medical reports from that time make little or no mention of psychoactive effects. In those days, people's expectations of cannabis were different. Either they did not get high from it because they did not expect to, or if they did, they paid it no attention and did not mention it to their doctors. It is expectation that leads us to associate our inner experiences of highs with the pharmacological effects of drugs.

The drawback of cannabis as a remedy is its extreme unpredictability. Its effects vary greatly from person to person. Doctors like drugs that have constant, reproducible effects, and they abandoned cannabis when they found more reliable, though sometimes more toxic, sedatives and antispasmodics.

Once, on reading through a nineteenth-century article on the medicinal properties of Indian hemp, I came across a line that caught my attention: "It is impossible to list the therapeutic indications for cannabis because the drug behaves homeopathically." What the writer meant, I think, is that cannabis treats individuals, not conditions. In the homeopathic conception, people get sick in unique ways; there are no "disease entities" apart from people. In my experience, this old observation about cannabis is quite true. Some people respond favorably to it and can use it to make themselves feel better when they are sick, no matter what they have. Other people do not respond favorably to cannabis and cannot use it at all as a remedy.

I know people who use marijuana successfully to treat headaches, insomnia, stomach and menstrual cramps, labor pains, and a variety of other minor ills. Some of them smoke it and some of them eat it. In general, they are people who like marijuana but do not use it too often and stay in good relationships with it. Just as marijuana triggers better highs when it is used less frequently, so also does it work better as a remedy when it is saved for occasions when it is really needed.

How can marijuana work for so many diverse conditions in some people? Such people are probably able to use marijuana as a tool for putting themselves in high states from which they can perceive the physical condition differently and thereby modify it. For example, headaches, like all diseases, are psychosomatic. That is, mind and body are both involved. (*Psychosomatic* just means "mind-body"; it does not mean "mind-caused" or "not physical.") The physical discomfort of headache captures the mind's attention, lending more energy to the physical problem in a vicious cycle. Shifting attention to a high, by any method, will break this cycle and permit the physical aspect of the disease to subside. People who respond favorably to marijuana have learned to use it to make this shift in attention.

Aside from these broad effects of marijuana in some people, the plant has certain specific pharmacological properties that may make it useful in the treatment of asthma, glaucoma, nausea, and spastic paralysis.

As a drug for asthma, marijuana has a paradoxical effect when smoked. It relaxes bronchial smooth muscle to permit greater airflow, but the irritation of the smoke may worsen the asthma. Which effect predominates depends on the individual. Some asthmatics report definite relief after smoking a joint, but others say the smoke precipitates fits of coughing. Ingesting the cannabis orally would be one way around this problem. Researchers are also experimenting with aerosol preparations of marijuana compounds that might give the relief without the irritation.

Glaucoma is a disease of the eye due to increased fluid pressure inside the eyeball. It is of unknown cause, and some forms of it lead to severe losses of vision. It is now treated by surgery and by drugs, but the drugs are often not very effective and have significant toxicity. Marijuana lowers intraocular pressure. How it does so is not known. Many glaucoma sufferers have found that their vision improves after smoking pot, and they prefer the side effects of marijuana to those of the conventional medicines. Research is underway to find preparations of cannabis that maximize this effect. At least one patient so far has forced the federal government to supply him with marijuana for his glaucoma.

As an antinausea drug, marijuana seems to have a place in modifying the toxic effects of the very poisonous drugs used in the chemotherapy of cancer. Many of these drugs produce violent nausea and vomiting within minutes of their injection. Marijuana, taken in advance, counteracts this toxicity, an effect discovered first by teen-agers with leukemia who happened to be potheads.

Marijuana may also be effective in the treatment of nausea from other causes, including motion sickness. Officials have not allowed researchers to test marijuana itself as an antinauseant. They have insisted, instead, on the use of chemically pure THC (tetrahydrocannabinol), the so-called active principle of the plant. THC does work when given orally, but as anyone familiar with medicinal plants knows, whole plants are safer and often better than concentrated chemicals extracted from them. I would like to see more research with marijuana and less with THC. And I am not in favor of the development of analogues of THC with no psychoactivity. With proper expectation, the psychoactivity of marijuana can be a powerful and beneficial psychosomatic influence on illness.

Spastic paralysis (or paralysis with increased muscle tone) results from interruption of central nervous system pathways to muscles. It occurs in birth injuries (cerebral palsy), spinal cord injuries, multiple sclerosis, stroke, and other conditions, and is an uncomfortable disability. Marijuana, by relaxing muscles, may be a specific treatment.

There are reports on other medicinal properties of cannabis, including antibiotic, antitumor, and antiepileptic effects of some of its derivatives. Other researchers have suggested using it as an appetite stimulant in old people and cancer patients. Here again, individual variability would likely be great and might discourage general use. Appetite stimulation from marijuana seems to be a consequence of expectation rather than a direct pharmacological effect.

If marijuana is to be used medicinally, it should be fresh and of good quality, as with any other medicinal plant. The therapeutic and psychoactive properties are in a resin that is concentrated in the flowering tops. The active compounds in this resin are soluble in oil but extremely insoluble in water. Therefore, infusions or decoctions of marijuana are not effective. Alcoholic tinctures are much more reliable but may not keep well. It is also possible to extract the active constituents in fat, for instance by boiling the plant in a mixture of butter and water, straining the mixture, and chilling it to separate the butter. (Several handbooks of marijuana give instructions for this method.)

Because of the insolubility of cannabis resin in water, it is absorbed unevenly from the gastrointestinal tract. This makes it hard to estimate doses of oral preparations and easy to take an overdose. One reason tincture of cannabis fell into disrepute in this century was the difficulty of establishing a standard dose for the average patient. Overdoses of marijuana are not dangerous, but they can be very uncomfortable. It is much better to err on the side of too little. In the absence of a standardized oral preparation, many users in our part of the world prefer to smoke the plant rather than eat it. Those who wish to use it orally will have to experiment with different forms and doses.

In discussing marijuana I have ignored the obvious fact of its illegality. Although laws on its possession and use are changing slowly, they still have a long way to go. Criminalization of marijuana has created large and unpleasant black markets (high-potency varieties now sell for $2000 a pound and more), promoted bad relationships with the drug, and seriously hampered good scientific research. Marijuana is much less toxic than many legal drugs, but many persons are afraid to use it medicinally because of its illegality and bad reputation. Abuse of marijuana is not uncommon today; to my mind it is a direct result of the approach our society has taken.

Sooner or later we will learn that plants with effects on the body and mind, such as marijuana, are what we make of them. Used intelligently and carefully they can help us. Used irresponsibly they can harm us. The problem is not to try to eradicate the plants (impossible) or stop people from using them (also impossible) but to teach the principles of safe interaction with them. Marijuana is certainly here to stay. I hope our relationships with it will improve.

11

IN THE LAND OF YAGÉ

No drug plant has excited more interest than *yagé*. A jungle vine whose ceremonial use by Indians was noted by early explorers of the Amazon basin, yagé is a powerful "remedy" among those tribes that still consume it ritually. It is also a pharmacological problem, imperfectly studied, and an exotic high sought out by drug users from all parts of the world.

In different areas of South America, this same drug is known by other names: *ayahuasca*, for instance, and *caapi*. To the botanist it is *Banisteriopsis caapi*, a vigorous and curious liana* of the Amazon forests, of relatively rare occurrence even in its home areas. The drug is prepared from the woody stem or trunk, which Colombian Indians call the *bejuco*. It is cut into manageable lengths, mashed by pounding with rocks, and boiled in water, usually along with one or more additives that vary from region to region. Then the plant material is discarded, and the liquid is cooked down to a concentrated extract. In eastern Colombia, some tribes prepare yagé as a simple cold water infusion.

Years ago, as a student in the Harvard Botanical Museum, I first saw pictures of *Banisteriopsis* and read much of the older literature about it. I knew that extracts of it commonly

---

* Lianas are huge climbing plants of tropical forests, one of the most characteristic features of "jungles." They spring from the forest floor, twine about the trunks of giant trees, and actually knit together the canopy of the forest. While they rely on trees only for support, some, like yagé, may grow so fast that they can kill their props by competing with them for light at the top of the canopy.

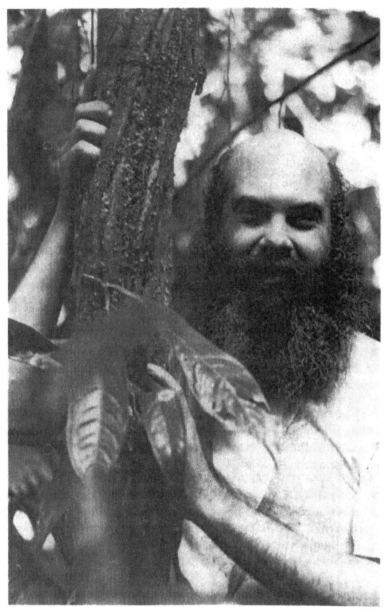

The author at the base of a specimen of yagé, *Banisteriopsis caapi*, in Colombia. (Silvia Patiño)

produce vomiting, diarrhea, and visions. Witch doctors credit it with the ability to confer telepathic powers, so that a yagé-intoxicated *brujo* ("witch") can communicate with people in other parts of the forest, if not the world, and also with the spirits of animals and plants. Telepathic powers are often attributed to the influence of magic plants by their users. (North American Indians say the same thing about peyote, for example). The association with yagé is especially strong, so much so that when German scientists first isolated the main alkaloid from the plant, they called it telepathine. (It is now known, less interestingly, as harmaline.) This alkaloid and others in *Banisteriopsis* belong to a family of drugs related chemically to such well-known hallucinogens as DMT and LSD. The pharmacological literature on harmaline is much less extensive than that on many other psychoactive drugs.

If scientific writings on yagé are inadequate, there is no lack of popular literature on the subject. In fact, a considerable mythology of yagé has accrued since the early 1950s. A major contributor to this body of folklore was William Burroughs, whose slim volume, *The Yagé Letters*, described his wanderings through the Putumayo Territory of southwest Colombia in search of the drug. The book is distinguished by a uniformly negative tone and, according to experts on the region, considerable misinformation. Nevertheless, it has become an underground classic and drawn thousands of young Americans and Europeans to the Putumayo. In a much more recent book, *Wizard of the Upper Amazon*, Manuel Córdova-Rios, a Peruvian healer, recounted his experiences as a child kidnapped by Amahuaca Indians and trained to be a future chief. His training consisted of frequent sessions with yagé, during which the natures of forest plants and animals were revealed to him in visions.

In addition to popular books, there exists an oral tradition of yagé tales in the drug subculture, not all of them very accurate. During a stay in the Haight-Ashbury in San Francisco in 1967, I was offered yagé by a vendor of unusual drugs. He called it the "tiger drug" because it was supposed to induce visions of jungle animals, especially of big cats, in all who took it. I thought this unlikely, but he assured me that "when Eskimos were given yagé in a laboratory, they saw visions of huge house cats, since they had never seen tigers." I pointed out (to no avail) that with the paucity of research on yagé, it was extremely improbable that anyone had done such an experiment. Also, I declined to buy any of his wares because it seemed to me that yagé could not be in very good condition by the time it reached San Francisco. (I should mention that Dr. Claudio Naranjo, a Chilean psychiatrist now living in Berkeley, reports in his recent book, *The Healing Journey*, that patients in Santiago given harmaline experimentally had visions of jungles and jaguars even though they had spent all of their lives in cities.)

Before I went to Colombia, I read more subjective accounts of the drug and talked with a few people who had taken it. Increasingly, I felt that I wanted to experience yagé firsthand, not only to satisfy my curiosity about its effects, which seemed highly variable, but also to see its use in various settings. Yagé is used in many different ways by many different groups of Indians in South America. I thought I might be able to draw some general conclusions about the interactions between social attitudes and effects of drugs by observing the uses of yagé among dissimilar tribes. It would be especially interesting to compare its effects in groups remote from the influence of Western civilization with those in more assimilated tribes.

I found myself on the trail of yagé almost as soon as I arrived in Bogotá. A Colombian botanist who had collected the plant in the Putumayo and was now organizing pharmacological research on it gave me much information, including the names of several brujos he thought I should visit. He also offered to take me to see a fine specimen of yagé growing not far from Bogotá. It seems he had brought cuttings of the plant from the Putumayo twelve years before and had planted them in the garden of a wealthy industrialist in a region where altitude and temperature create a climate similar to that of the plant's native area. In their new home the cuttings had thrived and were mature plants,

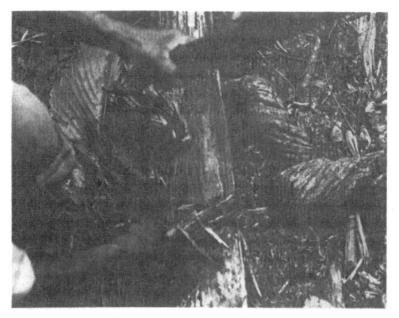

An Ingano shaman of the Caquetá Territory, Colombia, mashes lengths of yagé with a heavy stick. This pounding facilitates release of the hallucinogenic principles during cooking. (Diego León Giraldo)

possibly the only full-grown specimens of *Banisteriopsis* to be found outside of the Amazon basin.

We drove to this secret garden without delay, winding down from Bogotá's 8000-foot-high plain to warmer and sunnier lands. Our destination was a large country house surrounded by magnificient displays of flowering anthuriums, Birds-of-Paradise, and Torch Gingers — all perfectly groomed and obviously well cared for. Our host appeared and took us on a tour of the grounds. He seemed pleased to have the yagé on his property, and there was much joking about what would happen if the secret were discovered. (The consensus was that armies of hippies would descend to carry off the precious bejuco.) Returning from our tour, we examined the objects of our visit at leisure. Two massive lianas of yagé grew quite near the house in the midst of tropical lushness. A third was some distance off in the woods behind a greenhouse.

The plant nearest the house was enormous, its base a thick

aggregate of coiled trunks that soon branched out to entwine the tree it was growing on. Higher up, the tortuous woody stems, most as thick as a wrist, formed a crisscrossing network that obscured most of the trees. Everywhere, the small oval leaves of *Banisteriopsis* seemed to have better access to light than the leaves of its support. The liana was obviously at home in its new location. In fact, our host said it had grown so fast that it had already killed two nearby trees by competing with them so aggressively.

One of the lianas was in flower and fruit, and we collected a number of specimens to be mounted on herbarium sheets. The flowers are tiny and pink, quite inconspicuous against the giant growth of the whole plant. Then, with machetes, we hacked off a number of lengths of bejuco — sections of the woody stems about one foot long, from one to several inches in diameter. (The plant does not mind this kind of harvesting very much and quickly replaces what is taken.) These samples were needed for chemical analysis. In cross-section, the bejuco shows a characteristic pattern of the interior, more-vascular tissue. Indians refer to the lobes of this cross-sectional pattern as "hearts" and say that a liana is ready to use when it has seven or more hearts. Our specimens all had more than seven hearts, showing that the plant was fully mature. I chewed on a small piece of the woody tissue. It was quite bitter — an indication of its content of alkaloids. Growing in rich soil, with the lavish attention of gardeners, this yagé might be even more potent than the wild plant from which it was cut.

We left the garden with a bundle of yagé and our herbarium specimens. Seeing the living plant made me feel that I was close to my goal. The appearance of *Banisteriopsis* impressed me greatly; clearly, it is no ordinary plant. The potion that comes from it must be powerful stuff, I thought, not something to be taken casually. And I knew I would soon find out.

*

The Valley of Sibundoy in southwestern Colombia is a strange and beautiful world. Because of its natural isolation

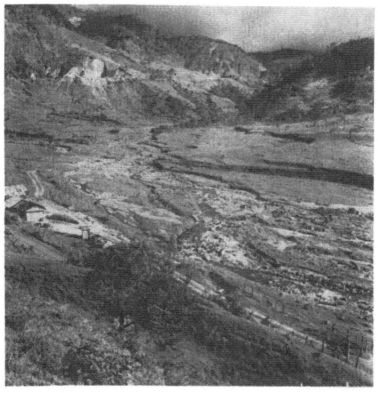

The Valley of Sibundoy, Putumayo Territory, Colombia. (R. E. Schultes)

by rugged mountains, the Indian villages within it have developed unique customs, particularly in regard to the use of plants. In fact, some of the plants themselves are unique, and one Colombian botanist I know says a man cannot really call himself a botanist until he has worked in Sibundoy.

An unpaved but good road leads to the valley from Pasto, the capital of the mountainous state of Nariño in the southwest corner of Colombia. Pasto is on the Pan American Highway and is near the border of Ecuador, where the three mountain chains that run through Colombia join to form the northern end of the *Cordillera de los Andes*, the backbone of peaks that runs the length of the western edge of South America. Leading east from Pasto, the road to Sibundoy climbs immediately through farmlands and slopes that are intensively cultivated despite their steepness. The land glows with a distinctive emerald-green color, a consequence of the richness of the volcanic soil. In a short time, the road climbs above 10,000 feet into a region of fog and peculiar low vegetation. Then, crossing the ridge, it drops quickly into a valley that holds a large and beautiful lake, the source of the Río Guamués, a tributary of the Putumayo.

After skirting the northern edge of this lake, the road climbs again, this time to nearly 12,000 feet, which brings it into a distinctive topographic zone known as *páramo*. Páramos are pockets of alpinelike vegetation that occur in certain parts of the tropics at elevations between 11,000 and 14,000 feet. They are favorite haunts of botanists because they contain a variety of species not found elsewhere. Colombia has a great many páramos, and they are popular sightseeing points because of their otherworldly beauty. Sightseers rarely stay for long, however, because the weather on a páramo, like the ground underfoot, is almost always soggy.

The páramo on the road to Sibundoy is small but lovely. The day I drove through it there was fog, mist, and drizzle. The ground was sodden and spongy, covered with many creeping plants of the heath or blueberry family and dotted everywhere with flowers. The most characteristic inhabitant of páramos is a relative of the sunflower — a tall plant with downy, silvery leaves and large yellow flowers (*Espeletia*) — and it was abundant on both sides of the road. Indians tie the large leaves around their foreheads to alleviate headache. As I continued on my way, the páramo ended abruptly. I was back in what botanists call "sub-páramo," the low, scrubby forest I had passed through on the previous ridge. Moments later, I crossed the border of the state of Nariño and entered the Territory of Putumayo. Spreading out before me, thousands of feet down, was the Valley of Sibundoy.

The Putumayo Territory is named for the Río Putumayo, a tributary of the Amazon and one of the mightiest rivers in South America. The Valley of Sibundoy is the source of this river, which begins here as a rushing brook. But the valley is not typical of the rest of the Territory, most of which is *tierra caliente*, hot country of tropical forests and rivers — in fact, the beginning of the Amazon basin. The valley is separated from the Amazon basin by a ridge of mountains to the east and is much higher and colder than the land on the other side. Its area is about 100 square miles, and as one winds down into it on the road from the west, it appears to be a fertile, flat basin, completely enclosed by mountains.

Four small towns and a few lesser settlements occupy the floor of the valley and are connected by the road. Santiago, the first town on the western edge, is the center of an Indian tribe known as the Ingas or Inganos, descendants of the ancient Incas, as their name suggests. Sibundoy itself, the largest community in the valley, is the tribal center of the Kamsas. Men of both tribes wear characteristic costumes that include several pounds of beads worn around the neck.

I arrived in the valley in the middle of "winter" — the season of heavy rain and clouds that runs from May through July. It rained a great deal while I was there. The sun peeked through the cloud cover occasionally, but almost always the weather was gray, damp, and chilly.

One of the first things I did on settling down in the town of Sibundoy was to call on Salvador, a Kamsa witch doctor who specializes in the preparation of yagé. Actually, the term *witch doctor* has no correspondence in Spanish. White scientists usually call men like Salvador *"brujos,"* but not to their faces, because the word has the same dark connotations as its English equivalent, "witches." The Spanish term for a medical doctor is *médico*, and some native practitioners insist on being addressed by it. A third term is *curandero*, or "healer," perhaps a more accurate designation for someone who can cure illness by unorthodox methods. Salvador, however, asks to be called a médico and has a certificate from a botanist at the National University in Bogotá announcing to whom it may concern that he is a skilled practitioner of herbal medicine, and, especially, an expert on the preparation and administration of yagé.

Now, yagé is a native of the hot country; it does not grow

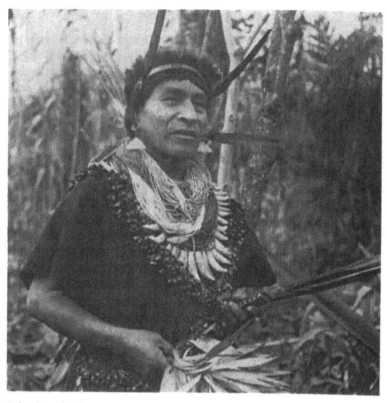

Salvador Chindoy, a Kamsa medicine man of Sibundoy, Colombia. (R. E. Schultes)

anywhere near the Valley of Sibundoy. Consequently, the Ingas and Kamsas who have learned its use have had to cross the mountains to the east and descend into the Amazon basin to study with men of tribes who live in the area where *Banisteriopsis* grows. When they want to use yagé, they must make the same long trip to get a supply of the bejuco to bring back to their valley.

Salvador lives with his family and animals in a thatched house not far from the town of Sibundoy. To get to it, one must tramp through fields that are quite wet in the rainy season and cross several mildly ticklish log bridges over small ravines. Eventually one reaches a sort of dense thicket of strange plants, in the middle of which is Salvador's house.

It is said that the inhabitants of the Valley of Sibundoy use a greater variety of intoxicating plants than any other people. Most of those plants grow right in Salvador's garden. Perhaps the most eye-catching are the Tree Daturas, or Brugmansias, relatives of our own Jimsonweed. They are mostly smallish trees, almost always in flower, and the flowers are quite spectacular: foot-long trumpets that hang straight down from the branches. Some are tubular and red, others flaring and white, with a thick, heady fragrance. All parts of these plants are intoxicating, if not actually poisonous, but local brujos use them regularly to induce altered states of consciousness. The Tree Daturas are known collectively as *borracheras*, a name that indicates their intoxicating power, because *borracho* is the Spanish adjective for "drunk." Like many other members of the Solanaceae, or nightshade family (such as Belladonna and Henbane), daturas contain mixtures of the so-called tropane alkaloids that cause delirium and amnesia. Two of these alkaloids, atropine and scopolamine, are used in orthodox medicine; scopolamine is the "twilight sleep" that is still used to make women amnesic for the experience of childbirth. Plants that contain tropane alkaloids are associated with witchcraft in many societies. A common sensation of people who consume them is that of flying through the air.

I have said that Salvador had Tree Daturas in his garden. Actually, his house seemed to be in the midst of a whole grove of them. It is most peculiar that in the Valley of Sibundoy and nowhere else Tree Daturas seem to be infected with a virus that makes them assume grotesque forms. At least, botanists assume the cause of these deformations is a virus because solanaceous plants are especially susceptible to viruses. (Tomatoes, tobacco, and potatoes, for example, are all attacked by virus diseases.) In Sibundoy these grotesque Tree Daturas breed true and are recognized by the Indians as distinct varieties with distinct pharmacological effects. Salvador had a number of them growing around his house in addition to the normal types.

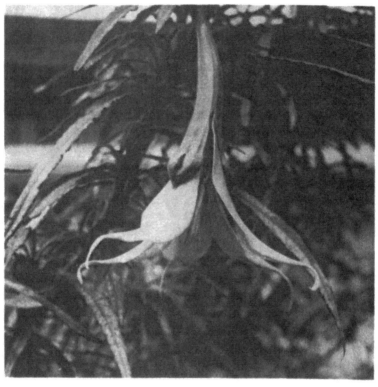

An atrophied form of Tree Datura in Sibundoy, Colombia. (R. E. Schultes)

The first time I entered the house, Salvador's wife was attempting to get a fire going in the middle of the earthen floor. A huge fire-blackened pot rested on some stones, and she was blowing on some glowing wood underneath it, trying to produce flames. The house was filled with smoke. It was mid-afternoon, but Salvador was curled up in bed, looking under the weather. With some effort he got up, explaining that he had taken yagé the previous evening with some visitors and was now tired. He says he is between sixty and seventy, but his face is youthful and of indeterminate age. He has an engaging smile. He speaks perfect Spanish with visitors, but converses among the members of his family in the Kamsa dialect.

Salvador told me that he was a famous médico, since people from all over came to see him, principally to take yagé. He showed me a book in which all of these visitors had recorded their names and addresses. Then he asked me if I would get him a document from the United States certifying him to be a médico and an expert on medicinal plants. It would have to have an official seal, he added. I said I would see. His request rubbed me the wrong way. After all, I hardly knew him, and if a medicine man is really a medicine man, why should he need certificates from the United States to prove it?

We drank several cups of *chicha*, a mildly alcoholic fermented mash of cornmeal, water, and raw sugar.* I told Salvador I was interested in seeing him prepare yagé and asked him what he made it from besides the bejuco. He said the only thing he added was the leaves of *Chagrapanga*. Chagrapanga, I knew from my reading, is a related species, *Diplopterys cabrerana*, whose leaves contain DMT (dimethyltryptamine) but none of the harmalines that are in *B. caapi*. Synthetic DMT, when available on the U.S. black market, is usually smoked (mixed with marijuana or mint leaves) and rarely injected. It cannot be taken by mouth because an enzyme in the human digestive tract inactivates it. But (as Indians have long known and pharmacologists have recently discovered) it is effective orally if mixed with yagé, because yagé contains substances that inhibit the enzyme. Consequently, Chagrapanga is never taken by itself but is always mixed with yagé, and it is one of the commonest additives to the potion. When I asked him why he added the Chagrapanga, Salvador replied: "To make the visions brighter" (*"Para brillar la pinta"*).

We decided that I should come back the next day to make and drink yagé. Salvador explained that the potion is pre-

---

* Chicha varies tremendously from locale to locale. Originally, it was made by masticating corn, spitting it into earthen vessels, and allowing it to ferment. The enzymes in saliva converted the starch to sugar, and yeasts in the air converted the sugar to alcohol. It is still made this way by tribes remote from Western influence. In Sibundoy today, sugar is added to a cornmeal-water mixture, and the chicha is drunk as soon as it is mildly carbonated and tangy.

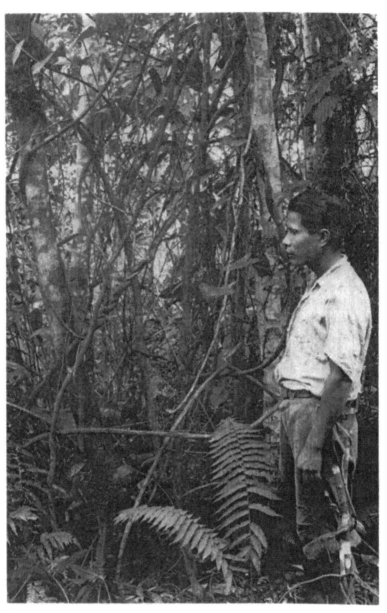

Chagrapanga, *Diplopterys cabrerana*, in the Amazon basin of Colombia. The leaves, containing DMT, are added to preparations of yagé to intensify the visionary effect. (R. E. Schultes)

pared in the afternoon and drunk only at night. Women may not be present during the preparation but may consume the finished drink. He told me I should not eat on the day of taking yagé and, particularly, should avoid milk. He then requested that I buy him some meat, coffee, salt, sugar, candles, and, most important of all, *aguardiente* for the ceremony. Aguardiente is an unaged whiskey distilled from sugar cane, strongly flavored with anise; it is the local firewater of South America. Since I like neither alcohol nor anise, I was not much looking forward to drinking it and wondered just how much of it we were going to use in this "ceremony."

I went back to the little town of Sibundoy to shop. It was a cold, gray afternoon. As usual, the streets were full of people doing nothing, mostly Indians but a fair number of hippies as well. This latter group was international: Americans, Europeans, Latin Americans, all with little or no money and yagé uppermost in their minds. Sibundoy, because it is the closest yagé center to the Pan American Highway, has been visited increasingly by hippies, many of whom have not the time or means to continue over the eastern mountains to the Amazon basin. Salvador's address book testifies that they have been coming for several years now. One effect has been that yagé has become good business for the brujos and médicos of the valley. For a fee, they will put on a yagé ceremony for you.

One of the surest ways to debase the ritual use of a drug is to begin selling the drug to strangers. Evidently this process had been going on in Sibundoy for some time, and what I was going to see would be a fairly debased ritual. I decided that a good way to gauge the degree of debasement would be to pay attention to the preparation of the drug. Most people who come to the valley pay their money and drink their yagé. I was glad I had asked Salvador to let me watch him make it, and I supposed his requests for groceries were the additional fee for this privilege. (I assumed he would want a few dollars' cash for the actual ceremony.) As a standard of comparison I had in mind a description of a yagé preparation that took place many years ago in the remote forests of Peru among a group of Amahuaca Indians as yet untouched by Western ways. These Indians made their drink from the bejuco of yagé and from the leaves of another plant, probably also Chagrapanga.

> . . . the serious preparations started, accompanied by almost continuous chanting. First the vine was cut into one-foot pieces with the stone ax and pounded on a flat stone with a large wooden mallet until it was well mashed . . . A layer of mashed vine pieces was then carefully arranged in the bottom of a large new clay pot. On top of this was laid a layer of the leaves in the shape of a fan . . . Then alternating layers of mashed vine and leaves were put in place until the pot was more than half full. Clear water from the stream was then added until the plant material was well covered.
>
> A slow fire was started under the pot and the cooking was maintained at a very low simmer for many hours until the liquid was reduced to less than half.
>
> When the cooking process was completed the fire was removed and, after cooling, the plant material was withdrawn from the liquid. After several hours of further cooling and settling, the clear green liquid was carefully dipped off into small clay pots, each fitted with a tight cover.
>
> The entire process took three days, being done with utter calmness and deliberation. The interminable chants accompanied each step, invoking the spirits of the vine, the shrub, and the other forest spirits.
>
> This carefully and reverently prepared extract provided the potion for many subsequent *ayahuasca* (i.e., yagé) sessions in the peaceful and secluded forest glade, sessions that progressed to incredible vision fantasies.*

Well, I thought, let us see how Salvador measures up.

When I went back to his *Datura*-surrounded house, it was raining steadily. By the time I got there, I was soaked. This time Salvador's son was present, Juan Pedro, a young man in his late twenties. I handed over the groceries, and Salvador immediately extracted the aguardiente, saying it

*F. Bruce Lamb, *Wizard of the Upper Amazon: The Story of Manuel Córdova-Rios*, 2nd ed. (Boston: Houghton Mifflin, 1975), pp. 32–33.

would be good for all of us to drink some. He poured shot glasses of the stuff. We all gulped it down in turn; it was even worse than I remembered from my last encounter with it a number of years before. Salvador was not satisfied with one round. He continued passing out the booze, usually serving himself two shots for every one given away, while Juan Pedro served up bowl after bowl of chicha. Outside, the rain kept up a steady patter. Inside, chickens ran around on the floor, and the fire went out, causing clouds of smoke — apparently a chronic problem in the wet season.

In a short time I was feeling pretty drunk, but the drinking went on with no signs of our doing anything about the yagé. Then Juan Pedro asked me if I had any marijuana on me. I told him I did not, which disappointed him, because he said many people who came told him how great marijuana was, but he had only smoked it once and had not gotten high on it. I managed to turn the conversation to yagé, and Salvador launched into a long series of anecdotes about the miraculous powers of the drug. (By the way, he never referred to it as a drug, but always as *el remedio* — "the remedy." However, the condition it produces is a *borrachera* or "intoxication.") There were stories of locating lost objects through yagé visions, solving crimes, and producing miracle cures. I listened to these stories with interest, but I have learned that witch doctors always have good raps about their products, and the stories are very much the same, whether the drug is peyote, yagé, magic mushrooms, or anything else (which may simply mean that the "effects" of the drug are really capacities of the mind in other states of consciousness).

Finally, when we had dispatched the bottle of aguardiente and my stomach was about bursting from the volume of chicha I had drunk, Salvador decided we could start making yagé. Happily the rain had let up, and a little bit of sun was even showing. We took wooden stools from the house and walked through the Tree Daturas to a little clearing partly sheltered by banana fronds. A large fire-blackened caldron was on the ground next to the ashes of an old fire. On a mat of banana leaves was a pile of the bejuco.

Salvador indicated that the first step was to strip off the

outer bark of the bejuco, and I set to work on that task with the blade of a pocket knife. The bejuco seemed neither very fresh nor very old. Looking at the cut ends, I noticed that it had the requisite number of "hearts" and therefore was mature enough for use. The bark came off easily. Meanwhile, Salvador had uncovered the caldron, which contained a mess of black, cooked leaves and mashed bejuco in a rusty brown liquid — the remains of the last batch of yagé. He poured the liquid into a bottle and fished out the spent leaves and stems. Then he seemed a bit confused and mumbled something about firewood that I did not catch.

The next step in the process was the mashing of the bejuco, a job that took considerably more energy because the stems — up to three inches in diameter — were tough wood. There was a smooth flat stone to lay them on and a heavy rock to pound with. I set to work, taking frequent rests. When I was finished and had an armload of mashed bejuco, Salvador announced that there was no firewood so that we would have to make this yagé without actually cooking it. Nor, apparently, was there any fresh Chagrapanga, because he began putting the old, black leaves back into the caldron with the freshly pounded bejuco. He then poured the liquid from the old brew into the pot, plus a little fresh water, and set about mashing everything together with a heavy stick. After about ten minutes, he felt the potion was finished and poured it into two empty aguardiente bottles; it was a muddy brown liquid. Then we walked back to the house.

In that moment I knew that I had no desire to spend more time with Salvador and certainly no interest in drinking his yagé. His preparation had turned out to be much sloppier than I could have imagined. I was not expecting a three-day production with interminable chants, but at least I wanted cooking. I doubted that Salvador's brown liquid had much potency except what might have been there from the previous batch, if that had been made properly.

It was now nearly dusk. Salvador suggested that I go off and return at nine to take the drug. "And don't forget to bring more aguardiente for tonight," he said. I was still a little wobbly from all the drinking I had done that afternoon; the thought of more anise-flavored alcohol did not make me feel better. I said good-bye and made my way back to the road.

To solidify my decision not to take yagé that night, I went back to Sibundoy and ate a large meal. My stomach had been crying out for something to soak up the remaining aguardiente and chicha. Shortly afterward the rain started again, this time in torrents. I doubt that I could have made it back to Salvador's house if I had wanted to.

I felt I had seen enough of yagé in Sibundoy. I decided I would leave the valley the next morning and head into the hot country, over the mountains to the little town of Mocoa, the capital of the Putumayo Territory. There, I hoped, the hippies would be fewer and the Indians a little more scrupulous about their yagé rites. Besides, the damp chill of winter in Sibundoy was getting to my bones. I longed to be somewhere where the chance of sunshine was a bit better.

I went to sleep that night listening to the heavy rain and thinking that the following night I would be warm.

But it was not to be.

*

The road from Sibundoy to Mocoa is one of the most dangerous in Colombia, especially in the wet season, when it is subject to frequent landslides. It is a narrow, unpaved track through the Cordillera Portachuelo, the last range of mountains before the Amazon basin. With luck the trip takes about three hours at an average speed of twenty miles an hour. The problem is that the road is heavily traveled, mainly by buses and huge trucks, since it is the only road connection from the interior of the Putumayo to the outside world. For most of its length the road is one way. By means of a system of checkpoints connected by telephone, large vehicles are detained until the way to the next checkpoint is clear. Small vehicles may pass but must be on guard for traffic coming head-on around the blind curves that crop up every few feet. During the rains, cars frequently go off the road and over the precipices below, and the route is often closed by slides.

For the first half-hour out of Sibundoy the road is two-way and usually in good condition as it crosses the final stretch of valley floor and begins the ascent into the Cordillera. On the Sunday morning I left, it had been raining hard for almost twenty-four hours. I had to ford deep flooded streams on the way up. Occasionally a whole section of road was gone, leaving little room for the car to squeeze between mountainside and cliff edge. Moreover, no traffic had come in the opposite direction since the previous afternoon, an ominous sign of what lay ahead.

I had a hitchhiker with me, a girl from California named Nancy who had been staying in Sibundoy with two friends, John and Lee. They were staying on there to take yagé with another brujo named Pedro; but she was more interested in warmth than yagé and wanted to reach Mocoa. I told her about my experiences with Salvador. She said her group had been to see him but decided not to take the drug with him because he wanted too much money — "a whole lot of groceries in addition to his fee." Pedro, it seemed, wanted only twenty pesos (one dollar) and the usual aguardiente.

When we reached the beginning of the one-way road, we learned that the way to the next checkpoint was blocked by three separate landslides. Because it was Sunday, there was not much action from the bulldozer teams whose job it is to clear the slides, but we thought we would wait to see what happened. As usual, it was a gray rainy day, even colder in the mountains than it had been in the valley. Over the next few hours, a line of trucks and buses built up behind us, the drivers and passengers all hoping to move onward. Occasionally the woman in charge of the little checkpoint station would call ahead to find out what was going on. The news was not good. It seemed there were fifteen landslides in all between our station and the last checkpoint, and, worse, the earthmoving machines were out of gas. We waited a little longer, then decided there was no hope of passage that day. Reluctantly, we headed back to Sibundoy.

Nancy suggested that I might want to talk to her friends about Pedro. We met John and Lee as we were pulling into town. They were just on their way to Pedro's house and said they would not mind at all if we came along. Unlike Salvador, Pedro lived right in town, but his house — wooden with a thatched roof — was more in the traditional Indian style than the tin-roofed adobe houses of his neighbors. He, too, had a gardenful of Tree Daturas, including some of the bizarre forms typical of the valley. Inside was the usual smoky fire and a veritable menagerie of chickens, dogs, cats, and dozens of birds roosting in the rafters. Pedro, also a Kamsa, was seated at a kind of desk heaped with papers and objects. He wore a felt hat and masses of beads around his neck and smoked continuously. (Indians throughout the Putumayo smoke a cheap brand of cigarettes called "Redskins" — *Pielroja* — whose trademark is the head of a North American Indian in full war bonnet.) Pedro had a young, kind face and a reserved, professional manner. He spoke with great deliberation.

It was late afternoon. John, Lee, Nancy, and I gathered around the fire. Pedro began to talk to us about yagé — more tales of its powers as a remedy for all ills. I asked him what went into his potion. He replied that he added Chagrapanga, borrachera (Tree Datura), and a mysterious fourth ingredient. His yagé was already made up; there would be no chance to watch the preparation. I was not very happy to hear about the borrachera. I am no lover of nightshade drugs, having had one experience with Jimsonweed that will last me a lifetime. Evidently, Pedro added a small amount of an infusion of the flowers of one type of borrachera. I asked him what the purpose of the Chagrapanga was and got the standard answer: "To make the visions brighter."

Pedro told us to come back at eight o'clock, not to eat anything (especially not milk), and not to forget the aguardiente. Before we left, he asked us to put our names in his book. He, too, has a little book and says that in the past few years people have come from "all parts" to learn about yagé from him.

We left the little house just after sunset. The rain had stopped, and I wondered whether I would be able to get through to Mocoa the next day — or whether I would be in any shape to try if I drank Pedro's potion. I was very aware that to drink yagé that night would be a violation of several resolutions I had made: not to drink yagé unless I had seen it made, not to take any *Datura*, and, in general, not to take a drug just because it happened to be available. But the day had been so discouraging and the prospect of a night in Sibundoy with nothing to do was so dismal that I decided to go ahead and violate all of my resolutions. John and Lee felt they had "good rapport" with Pedro. Nancy said she would happily keep us company but had no desire to take the remedy.

And so at eight o'clock, aguardiente in hand, we trooped back to Pedro's house, which was now quite dark except for a candle burning on his desk. Pedro was still at the desk, just as we had left him, but beside him, stretched out on a rough bed, head swathed in bandages, was an Ingano patient. He remained there the whole night, and Pedro frequently conversed with him, though we never found out exactly what his problem was. It was somehow reassuring to see that Pedro actually had patients. In fact, minutes later, another man came to consult him, apparently about a problem of excess drinking. Pedro gave him advice in slow, measured tones while smoking incessantly and spitting on the floor under his desk. This man was told to return at six the following morning.

We sat around in silence for what seemed a long time until, at last, the church bell tolled nine o'clock. With great solemnity Pedro began to drink and serve shots of aguardiente. He explained it was necessary to facilitate the effect of yagé. I gritted my teeth and gulped it down. Including the patient in bed, all of us but Nancy drank three rounds of it. Then, after another silent period during which I began to feel high on the alcohol, Pedro fetched a bottle of brown liquid and poured it into a bowl. He studied the liquid for a time, then began to perform various rites over it that seemed to be purifying in intent. They included blowing cigarette smoke onto it, shaking a bunch of dried leaves rhythmically around all sides of the bowl, and, finally, chanting. Pedro's yagé chant was a half-whispered, half-whistled tune, quite melodic, sometimes wordless, sometimes with words. When it was over, he filled a small tumbler (about four ounces) to the brim from the bowl, drank it down in one swallow, and followed it with a shot of aguardiente. Then he asked us to wait for him for a moment.

Again we sat in silence. After many minutes, Pedro filled the tumbler again and handed it to me. I took it, thought to myself, For science, and drained it down. It was, as I expected, terribly bitter (though not so bitter as peyote), and the follow-up shot of aguardiente was welcome for the first time. I handed the empty tumbler back to Pedro and he proceeded to pour out the same dose for John and Lee.

More silence. Pedro asked us to let him know when we felt something and said we could have more if we wanted but should first wait a bit. After only ten minutes, I began to feel something very definite. It started as a feeling of warmth and strangeness in my stomach, spreading rapidly to my chest and arms. This sensation increased rapidly, soon changing into a kind of thrill or vibration in all my muscles. These feelings were pleasant, seeming to represent a tremendous energy flowing through my body. At the same time I felt very clear-headed and euphoric. My companions evidently felt nothing at all yet.

Over the next few minutes, I began to enter a state of consciousness somewhere between waking and dozing, with the physical sensations of energy and vibration continuing unchanged. In this reverie I had many thoughts that seemed inspired. Whenever I opened my eyes, Pedro was in the same position at his desk, his face illuminated by the candle, looking intently, sometimes at me, sometimes at the others. I am not sure how much time went by. The next thing I became aware of was that John was sick. He stumbled from the room to an outhouse and we could hear him retching violently for what seemed hours. Lee said he still felt nothing.

John came back looking pale and shaky. Moments later, he rushed from the house again and was seized by another endless bout of retching.

Then Pedro went out and apparently vomited also. He came back quickly and resumed his former position. I am not sure how much I was influenced by all this audible evidence of sickness. Nor can I say there was a clear-cut end to my experience of feeling exhilarated and well. I only know that I began gradually to feel unwell. At first I entertained the vain hope that I could avoid getting sick by an effort of will. I lay down on the floor on my back, took deep breaths, and tried to ignore the growing nausea that welled up from my insides. The vibrations in my muscles kept going but now were annoying rather than pleasant because they made me feel that my body was in the grip of something I could not influence. I felt no inclination to vomit, but I was aware of intestinal cramps and knew I would have to move my bowels. But getting up and going outside seemed an impossibility.

Eventually, my bowels insisted. I staggered to my feet and lurched toward the door, out into the cold night. I had almost no control over my legs and avoided sprawling on the ground only by running into a tree. Every movement produced waves of agonizing nausea. Somehow I got to the outhouse. It was raining again — a cold drizzle. I saw John lying in the mud, holding his stomach and still retching. There was nothing left inside him to come up, but he could not stop the spasms. Inside the outhouse, my bowels emptied themselves of everything they contained. If nothing else, yagé is surely the most powerful purgative I have ever encountered. Unfortunately, the purge did not make me feel better, and when I crawled out into the night I could do nothing but lie helplessly on the wet ground. Even thinking about moving set off new waves of sickness.

I now began to have visions, although my awareness was so dominated by the reality of being sick that I could not pay careful attention to them. These visions were like waking dreams. There was much motion, many scenes of people and places. I am sorry to say there were no jungles or jaguars, nor any telepathic news bulletins of distant events. The visions simply went on in one sphere of my consciousness, while cold-night-sickness-and-John-retching occupied another more vivid sphere. I knew I should try to get back to the house, which at least was dry and warm, but I just could not move.

Nancy was a great comfort during this period of misery. She tried very hard not to say "I told you so," and made John and me feel that at least someone cared. (Pedro seemed to have abandoned us to our fate, and Lee was still complaining that he felt nothing.) She tried to help me up, but the effort made me worse, and I collapsed again on the cold ground. She sat beside me for a while, talking about California, and, though I could not really concentrate on what she was saying, her voice was soothing. I do remember her telling me that she once watched two people take LSD for the first time. They both became sick, and she decided never to have anything to do with psychedelic drugs. She was certainly getting a lot of reinforcement in that decision now, I thought.

Quite suddenly I had a violent spasm in my stomach and vomited up a small quantity of intensely bitter liquid flavored with that awful anise of aguardiente. I could feel the taste through my whole body. Then I had a brief period of unproductive retching. It was quite painful, and I felt a surge of compassion for poor John, who was still doing it. After another indeterminate period, Lee came out. He now had diarrhea, which was something to write home about, but insisted he felt no other effects.

I was cold and wet in addition to being sick. The visions continued, although I still could not watch them. Finally, Lee half-carried me into the house, and I lay down in a hard bed. I did not sleep at all during the night, owing to the stimulation of the drug. Gradually, the worst of the symptoms subsided. Pedro crawled into bed with his patient and the two of them kept up a lively conversation. The fire was out, and the temperature of the room dropped. Lee, John, and I huddled together under a single, thin blanket trying to keep warm.

Well before dawn, several roosters began crowing for all they were worth. Then the first light showed, and Pedro's wife started the fire up. Promptly at six, Pedro's other patient arrived. Pedro came over to the bed in which the three of us were lying and blew incense on us. Then he shook his bunch of leaves over us and chanted a bit. He said that would end the effect of the yagé. We got up and went over to the fire. I felt thoroughly cleaned out — a bit weak but otherwise all right. I longed for a glass of orange juice and could not wait to get away from Pedro's house to get one. Just then Pedro produced another bottle of aguardiente and said we had to drink some to cleanse the yagé from our systems. I cannot describe the revulsion I felt at the thought of drinking aguardiente at that hour after that night. I pleaded an upset stomach. But Pedro insisted. When I said I really couldn't, he began to complain that I was not following his instructions. So I ended up swallowing two shots of the stuff and wishing I were dead. When he gave me a third, I held it in my mouth and spit it out in the corner while pretending to look for my jacket.

Pedro told me to remember that some people got sick the first time they tried yagé and that the cure was to take more. His last words to me were to be sure to tell people about him and send him more customers. I paid him his twenty pesos and left the house, feeling that an ordeal was behind me. I had certainly experienced a fully debased yagé ritual, I thought — light on the ceremony, heavy on the aguardiente. People in town said that a flotilla of trucks and buses had arrived from Mocoa during the night, meaning the road was open at last, and after having my orange juice, I said goodbye to Sibundoy with much pleasure.

*

The next-to-last checkpoint on the one-way road from Sibundoy to Mocoa is called *Mirador* ("Lookout"). It looks out on a spectacular view: the sheer drop of the eastern edge of the

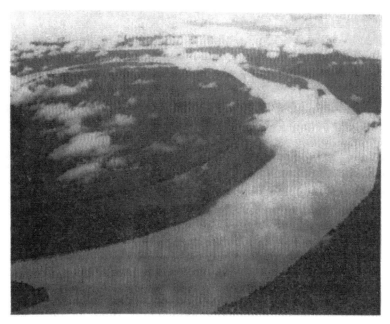

Río Putumayo, Colombia, on its way to join the Amazon. (R. E. Schultes)

Cordillera Portachuelo, with the road falling thousands of feet in narrow switchbacks and the panorama of the Amazon basin stretching out to the distant horizon. Here begins the most dangerous part of the road — a steep, twisting descent that leads, finally, out of the mountains and into the land of forest and river. It is a great relief when the last checkpoint is passed and one can accelerate a bit without fear of falling off a mountain.

Of course, it was still winter when I arrived, meaning more rain and gray skies, but there were sun and rainbows, too. When the sun is out, with puffy cumulus clouds dotting a bright blue sky, the Putumayo seems a very good place to be. Yagé is much talked about here, along with the famous *machaca*, a mythical beetle whose bite is supposed to be the most powerful aphrodisiac known: death within twenty-four hours, goes the tale, unless one makes love. A recently published government booklet designed to promote tourism in the Putumayo Territory boasts about the machaca and says also that the colors and images of native handicrafts are invented "by taking doses of hallucinogens like yagé." It goes on to hint at the existence of hallucinogenic mushrooms in the Territory as well.

Not surprisingly, this kind of advertising has brought numbers of hippies to the Putumayo and, in addition, has given impetus to the commercialization of yagé. In fact, in Mocoa itself and in all the sleazy communities along the road to the busy town of Puerto Asís on the Río Putumayo, yagé "priests" abound who sell the drug and its rites for money and aguardiente. The fee is usually lower than in Sibundoy. I was not surprised to find this degree of commercialization but hoped to see something to do with the drug that was a bit more inspiring than what I had found in Sibundoy.

A few days after getting to Mocoa, I kept a date with a witch doctor a few miles from town to prepare yagé with him. His name was Ambrosio, an Indian of the Mocoa tribe who lived in an isolated house above the banks of the Río Rumiyaco. Like most of the rivers in the area, the Rumiyaco is a roaring torrent, fresh out of the mountains, especially high at this time of year. It was raining hard the morning I went to cook yagé with Ambrosio, and the path along the river was slippery mud. It skirted fields of sugar cane and occasional patches of pineapple, then crossed the river on a log bridge. On the other side I had to scramble up a muddy bank, walk through wet fields, and then struggle up a long hill. The house was a rickety wooden frame, high above the ground on stilts, thatched over with palm fronds. Ambrosio and his son Carlos were there along with another Indian, who, Ambrosio said, was sick with fever. They all seemed a bit drunk, although it was early morning.

Ambrosio does some carpentry, but he is more interested in yagé than wood. He has both yagé and Chagrapanga growing near his house. When I had visited him the previous afternoon, he had said we could cook up a batch from scratch. Ambrosio laughs at nearly everything that happens or anything anyone says to him. This morning things seemed to strike him especially funny.

I had brought along the expected offering of aguardiente. Once I had established that we were not going to drink it off immediately, we decided the first order of business would be to collect the leaves of Chagrapanga. Accordingly, Ambrosio, with a woven basket on his back, Carlos, with a machete, and I, with nothing, trudged out into the pouring rain, down a muddy hillside into a tangle of vegetation where Chagrapanga was to be found. The plant (or plants — it was hard to tell in such dense undergrowth) seemed to be a shrubby, woody vine with many large smooth leaves. Carlos and I ripped off handfuls of them and stuffed them into Ambrosio's basket. When the basket was nearly full, we left the site and marched farther on in the same direction.

Presently we came to a cliff and, climbing down it, reached the bank of the Rumiyaco, where there was a sort of *ramada* — an open, thatched hut that seemed to be used for cooking yagé. In the middle of it was a fire pit full of ashes, and piled up to one side was a huge stack of wood, mostly trunks of small trees about six feet long. Getting a fire started was not easy. We had only a few matches among us, Ambrosio's lighter was out of fluid, and everything was sodden. We assembled a stack of logs, together with much kindling, and got some sparks going but couldn't seem to produce flames. Ambrosio found all of this immensely funny. After much work, the fire roared to life, and we arranged the logs so that they could be pushed into the pit from different directions as they were consumed. Carlos took a huge, fire-blackened kettle to the river, filled it with water, and set it on some rocks over the fire. Into it went the Chagrapanga leaves from the basket.

"Now we get the yagé," said Carlos. "We go up." And up we went, up a mountainside of pure mud, slipping, sliding, and sloshing. Ambrosio laughed all the way, especially loudly whenever he fell into the mud. After an endless climb, we got to the top and turned off the path into a dense woods. Carlos hacked open a path for us, and after a good trek, we came to a place where several large trees had fallen. Twined all about these fallen trees and completely tangled with the neighboring brush were the huge woody stems of *Banis-*

teriopsis caapi. We had reached Ambrosio's yagé grove.

Carlos set about chopping off lengths of bejuco and cutting them into one-foot sections. I loaded them into the basket of Ambrosio, who was now giggling quietly to himself. When the basket was nearly full, we retraced our steps and began the descent of the mudslide, which reactivated Ambrosio's full-blown hysterics. I thought we would go immediately to the pot to add the bejuco, but Carlos said, "Let's leave it here and go have some aguardiente first." I saw no good coming of this decision, but while I was considering how to object, Ambrosio threw down the basket, and he and Carlos went off in the direction of the house. I followed through a field of ankle-deep mud.

This time I had the sense to decline aguardiente right from the beginning (I said it was bad for my stomach) and merely watched while Carlos, Ambrosio, and the sick friend killed the whole bottle. The rain increased steadily, to the delight only of a family of ducks that padded around outside the house. Ambrosio and Carlos were soon so drunk that they could hardly stand and wore glazed expressions. At every opportunity, I urged them to resume the job of cooking the yagé, but the alcoholic inertia was terrific. Finally, finally, we all started off into the downpour to collect the basket of bejuco. Ambrosio's laugh had become a drunken cackle. He got quite lost trying to get back to the ramada. It was with some difficulty that we reached the cliff, got down it, and eventually came out on the right spot. Of course, the fire had gone out. Starting it was only slightly easier than before.

"That's Chagrapanga," Carlos told me, pointing to the kettle and weaving back and forth. He repeated this statement about thirty times in the next hour, not being able to think of anything else to say. "What does the Chagrapanga do?" I asked. "It makes the visions brighter," Ambrosio replied, as if that were the most hilarious joke in the world. Then we began scraping the bejuco, pounding it with rocks, and adding it to the caldron. Carlos stirred the mixture with a long paddle. Now that it no longer consisted of just Chagrapanga, he had to think of a new thing to say to me. He quickly hit upon, "*¿Cómo le parece, Doctor?*" ("How does it look to you,

Doctor?''), which he asked me every few minutes for the duration of the cooking.

For the next hour and a half, we sat on logs, took turns stirring the brew and rearranging the logs in the fire, and listened to the downpour. Ambrosio laughed. Carlos kept asking me how it looked. (*"Muy bien"* was the only thing I could think of to answer, but it seemed to please him.) The pot boiled vigorously. After about two hours of cooking in all, Ambrosio thought the rusty-brown soup was done. We poured the liquid into another pot, discarded the leaves and bejuco, then returned the liquid to the large kettle and quickly boiled it down to about a quart, just enough to fit into an empty aguardiente bottle.

It was now late afternoon, and, miraculously, the rain stopped. Ambrosio asked if I wanted to drink the yagé that night. No, I told him, I would rather take it with me. That was fine with him. This preparation of yagé was a considerable improvement over Salvador's in Sibundoy, but I did not feel drawn to drink it in an atmosphere so thick with alcoholic haze. As it turned out, I never got to drink it. The stuff fermented within a week, producing a luxuriant growth of evil-looking fungus.

I regret to say that, although I looked quite hard in the Putumayo, I did not find any yagé men who inspired greater confidence.

*

Debasement of Sibundoy Indian culture is a sad and logical result of national development and is a model for the erosion of traditional life throughout South America. Not long ago, the Valley of Sibundoy had some of the most interesting uses of psychoactive and medicinal plants in the world. Today, alcoholism is replacing the ceremonial use of safer drugs.

If anything, the situation is worse in the interior of the Putumayo. The problem there is oil — huge deposits of it, now being pumped out of the ground, refined, and transported over the Andes to the Pacific. Texaco has built a refinery town in the middle of the jungle. It has been a disaster for the physical and social ecology of this section of the Amazon basin. The prospects of fast money drew thousands of un-savory characters to the seedy towns of the Putumayo and stimulated a great bout of road building and development.

Of course, it is the Indians who have suffered most from these changes. Symbolic of the destruction of their ways of life is the introduction of distilled alcohol. Amazonian tribes have their own traditional fermented beers (chicha), which serve them well, but they cannot learn to control the white man's firewater. I learned the hard way that when I want to see something of the positive uses of psychoactive plants by South American Indians, it is not worth visiting tribes who have access to spirits.

Around Mocoa I saw a number of other *yageros*, local yagé priests recommended to me by residents of the area. All of them turned out to be drunks. Finally, I made an arduous journey through Kofán territory near the Ecuadorian border to find a shaman removed from the pernicious influence of encroaching civilization. I left El Rojo at the end of the road system in the care of a friend, traveled a long way by motor launch and canoe, then walked through the forest over a dif-ficult trail. When I arrived at the hut of the shaman, he was away, due back in a few days. An Indian girl said I could stay, and I strung up my hammock in the hut. For several days I fought off sandflies and drank in the beauty of the forest and a swift river that ran nearby.

When the shaman returned, he told me he was sorry that he had no time to prepare yagé anymore. He was now travel-ing all the time, trying to get the Kofán people to sign peti-tions demanding reparations from the territorial govern-ment for damage done by the oil company. Even in this remote spot, he said, the noise of Texaco's helicopters had driven fish and game from the rivers and jungles, so that his people could no longer satisfy their needs by hunting.

*

My travels in the land of yagé were disappointing but educa-tional. They showed me that traditional peoples do not auto-matically form good relationships with psychoactive plants.

In a stable traditional culture, that ideal can be a reality, but under the pressure of change, Indians, like the rest of us, are capable of using drugs unwisely.

I remain interested in yagé and hope someday to find a place where people still use it reverently and do not drink aguardiente. I am not very eager to take it again until I find such a place. There are still regions of the Amazon far from roads, hippies, and oil refineries, where yagé rituals exist. I will visit them when I can.

12

IS HEROIN AS DANGEROUS
AS WHITE SUGAR?

SUGAR CANE is a constant feature of American tropical landscapes. In the continental United States, most people consume large quantities of white sugar, chemically pure sucrose that is extracted and refined from cane juice, but few have seen the plant growing. Being around sugar cane fields made me more aware of the different ways we can use this plant and gave me some new ideas about white sugar.

The most direct and natural way to eat sugar cane is to cut a length of the fresh stalk, peel it, and chew on it, sucking the sweet juice and spitting out the fiber. Children in the hot country of Latin America are avid gnawers of cane. For my taste, the reward of the fresh juice does not quite make up for the disagreeableness of a mouthful of fiber; I prefer to get my sugar in another form. In Cuernavaca, Mexico, a popular juice bar sells fresh *jugo de caña* (cane juice, pressed from the stalks and dispensed from a spray cooler) as a health drink, advertising it as "rich in minerals and vitamins." In other places I have seen sidewalk vendors with portable presses sell glasses of the same freshly squeezed juice. It is a grayish-green, watery liquid, sweet, of course, but insipid in flavor. It has a faintly unpleasant back taste that some people dislike. A slice of lime improves it greatly.

If cane juice sits in a warm place for a day or two, it turns brown, tangy, and alcoholic. It is then *guarapo*, a popular drink of workers at cane-processing plants and a home brew of hot-country Indians that is little known in the cities. At its

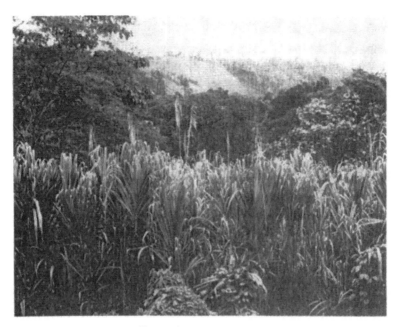

Sugar cane, *Saccharum officinarum*, is a giant grass native to Asia, now cultivated throughout the tropics. The stalks contain a sweet juice from which sugar is extracted. (Bob Harris)

best, guarapo is like a good hard cider, slightly sparkling, sweet, and refreshing. But what happens to the fresh juice of sugar cane on its way to becoming the pure white powder we are all familiar with?

The first step in the process is concentration. The cane juice is boiled down, often in large copper-lined vessels over open wood fires, to drive off excess water as steam. As the juice reduces in volume, it darkens and acquires a strong, characteristic flavor. When it is concentrated to a syrup of the proper density, it is poured into molds, where it quickly crystallizes into blocks of raw sugar known as *panela*.

Panela bears little resemblance to anything Americans know as "brown" or "raw" sugar. What is sold as "light brown" and "dark brown" sugar in U.S. grocery stores is really refined white sugar colored and flavored by the addition of molasses. The "raw" sugars sold at such high prices by health food stores are prepared in the same way: that is, they are processed only one step further than white sugar.

Panela is the true and only raw sugar. Sold all over tropical Latin America, in supermarkets as well as Indian markets, it comes in many shapes, from blocks the size of building bricks to large hemispheres and cones ("sugar loaves"), and a variety of colors, from dark brown to light russet. Although panela is widely available and widely consumed in Latin America, it is only a runner-up to white sugar in total sales and uses. Even most cane workers and Indians seem to prefer to use white sugar as their ordinary sweetener, saving panela for special pastries, candies, and beverages. I have often seen cane workers adding white sugar to their coffee while blocks of panela are crystallizing a few feet away. Similarly, most North Americans have come to rely on white sugar for ordinary uses, saving brown sugar for special dishes where its different flavor is desired.

The only way I can describe the taste of panela is to say that its differentness from white sugar is much more pronounced. Many North Americans who try panela for the first time do not like it. Even people who do like it, like it in things where its flavor is diffused and modified. Sometimes I like a taste of straight panela, especially out of a mold where it is cooling, but I never care to eat more than a lick from the end of a finger. It is to remove these disagreeable flavors that panela is subjected to further processing.

If raw sugar is dissolved in fresh water, boiled down to a syrup again, and cooled, it crystallizes out lighter in color and flavor than the liquor left behind. This liquor, when concentrated, is molasses. It contains the impurities that color and flavor cane syrup, along with some sugar. By a series of fecrystallizations and centrifugations, sugar can be made completely free of these additional compounds. As by-products, various grades of molasses are collected, ranging in taste from those that are useful as distinctive sweeteners in their own right to those so strong that they are fit only as feed supplements for animals. (Much molasses is fermented and distilled into rum.)

White sugar, then, is the pure sweet principle isolated

from the natural context of flavors in which it occurs in cane juice. Those flavors, concentrated and minus most of the sweet principle, do not taste very good. Because of its non-naturalness, white sugar is shunned by persons who follow diets rich in natural foods. Some advocates of natural foods cannot talk about white sugar without becoming irate. Here, for example, is the opening paragraph of a tract called "The Sugar Story," distributed in U.S. health food stores: "No organic merchant sells white sugar or any products containing white sugar because it is a foodless food. It is 99.95% sucrose and when taken into the human body in this form is potentially dangerous. It is touted as an energy food, but such propaganda is misleading, for there is ample evidence that white sugar robs the body of B vitamins, disrupts calcium metabolism, and has a deleterious effect on the nervous system." The author goes on to denounce brown and raw sugars as "phony": "Having done a thorough personal investigation, I can assure you that brown sugar is nothing more than white sugar wearing a mask." He also paints grim pictures of sugar refineries, conjuring up images of huge filtration units "filled with charred beef bones" that are certain to horrify patrons of health food stores.

I find it difficult to evaluate this sort of polemic because I am of two minds on the subject. On the one hand, I do not know of "ample evidence" that white sugar robs the body of B vitamins, disrupts calcium metabolism, harms the nervous system, or does anything else of comparable awfulness. At the same time, I am in sympathy with the idea that more-natural substances are inherently less dangerous than less natural ones.

Some years ago, at a drug symposium in Michigan, I heard a remark that seemed outrageous. A long-haired representative of the counterculture, arguing against the value judgments society has made about some drugs, told an audience of schoolteachers that he and his friends thought white sugar was "addicting and more dangerous than heroin." The audience was suitably shocked. Of course, it is not possible to compare the two: One is an intoxicant, the other a food (or nonfood, to some); one is put into the nose, lungs, or veins, the other into the mouth and stomach. But let us see if there is anything to learn from an analogy drawn between two pure chemicals that are far removed from their natural sources.

Heroin is a synthetic derivative of morphine, which itself is only one of twenty-two alkaloids in the latex of the opium poppy. Its relationship to opium as an intoxicant does seem to me analogous to the relationship between white sugar and the panela of Latin America. In both cases the pure white powders are the results of attempts to separate out a single component of something that is naturally complex. The motivation for this processing is the craving for a more pleasurable experience: for stronger sweetness in the sugar eater, for a stronger rush of intoxication in the addict. But heroin is not a good substance for most people to be involved with. Its use tends to get out of hand. This is so because of its nature: it is too easy to use too much of it too much of the time. Opium is a gummy, dark resin that cannot be injected because it is impure. Pure white heroin can be pumped into veins as fast as one can obtain it.

Intravenous heroin is so reinforcing that few addicts are able to appreciate other sorts of highs. All they can talk about is the "rush" of heroin, how nothing else compares. It is also a short-acting drug, which creates practical problems for those who would like to create heroin maintenance programs for addicts. Clients of such programs would have to live in or come in several times a day for shots. By contrast, oral opium is long-acting and much less liable to abuse. Taken in excess, it causes severe nausea that deters overuse. (Smoked opium does not have this built-in safeguard.) I think addicts who are motivated to change their drug habits could get from it what they like, learn to use it in a moderate and stable fashion, and be able to live away from the treatment facility. I would very much like to see an experimental trial of oral opium maintenance for addicts, since I think it would produce better results than treatment with either methadone or heroin, which are refinements and distortions of the pleasure-giving element of the poppy plant.

The real trouble with white sugar is that, like heroin, it is too reinforcing. Most of us are sugar addicts who would have great difficulty going through a single day with no sugar whatever. A great deal of our food contains hidden sugar, added by manufacturers to make it taste right to us. This dietary excess is certainly the principal cause of dental caries. It might also be an important factor in our tendencies toward obesity and cardiovascular disease. Also, I think there is some evidence that premature deposition of cholesterol in human arteries is correlated with a disorder of sugar metabolism rather than one of fat metabolism.

Evolutionarily, it makes sense that we are so attracted to sugar. Sugar is instant energy, which could mean survival. In prehistory, when our sweet tooth evolved, sugar was rare. It occurred in fruit and an occasional honeycomb, and our ancestors who developed cravings for those tastes had a survival advantage. Evolution, however, did not anticipate a day when sugar in great quantity would be available at every turn. The reinforcing quality of sugar, once so logical, now works against us. I am certain that people would eat less sugar if the only cane product they could get were panela. It is much easier to be a regular, heavy consumer of the refined product, just as it is much easier to get hooked on heroin than on opium.

Perhaps, then, the problem with refining natural substances into white powders is that we lose in the process certain signals that encourage us to use potentially harmful things in moderation. The disagreeable taste that builds up as cane juice is boiled down might be a clue telling us not to seek sweetness in concentrated form beyond a certain point. The nausea produced by opium should suggest to poppy lovers that they limit their intake and dosage.

Because the process of refining, if carried too far, leads to the creation of pure substances that may be much harder to control than natural substances, some people conclude that processing itself is wrong, that we should consume only wild, raw, unprocessed foods. I believe that man can improve on nature and should not cease trying to make natural things better. The cultivation of fruits and vegetables to produce superior varieties is an example of good tampering with nature (provided the qualities selected for development are goodness and flavor rather than uniformity of size and resistance to shipping). Similarly, the preparation of foods for the table can enhance natural qualities without destroying them.

There must be a middle ground between the synthetic foodlike products that occupy more and more space in supermarkets and the faddist's diet of raw fruits and vegetables. In my own diet I use honey, some molasses and maple syrup, and a little white sugar when I want neutral sweetness without a special flavor. I do not avoid white sugar as a poison or nonfood, but I do regard it as more liable to abuse than any other sweetener. Also, I look forward to being again in areas of the world where I can buy panela, the true raw sugar of the tropics.

13

THE GREEN AND THE WHITE: COCA AND COCAINE

SCENE: The international arrivals section of Eldorado Airport, Bogotá, Colombia, one night in mid-December 1973. Passengers who have cleared customs enter the long hall of airline ticket counters through double doors and are met by porters, friends, and taxi drivers. The author is sitting nearby, waiting to meet someone.

Enter: Through the double doors a man and a woman in their mid-thirties, Americans, nonhippies. The woman wears a long summer dress, the man Bermuda shorts — inappropriate clothes for Bogotá's 8000-foot altitude. They might have just stepped off a plane from Miami. Both of them seem agitated. They look around, not sure where to go. The woman sees the author and walks up to him.

WOMAN (breathlessly): Excuse me, do you speak English?
AUTHOR: Yes.
WOMAN: Well, we just got off the plane this minute. Can you tell us where we can get some cocaine right away, tonight?

*

When I first came to Bogotá in 1965, Eldorado Airport was less fancy but more hospitable. As soon as passengers cleared customs they were ushered to a round pavilion and served free cups of delicious coffee, compliments of the national coffee growers' association. Today, free samples of cocaine might be more to the point. A great many visitors to Colombia have cocaine uppermost in their minds. It is said that the amount of money involved in its illegal export to the North makes it at least as important economically as coffee.

It is not surprising that many of the cocaine seekers who come to Colombia are Americans. The popularity of cocaine in the United States is at an all-time high. More important, its use has now invaded the world of the middle classes, just as marijuana use did, starting a decade ago. One consequence of this change is a growing campaign on the part of middle-class lawyers, doctors, and educators to convince the public in general and judges in particular that cocaine is much less harmful than our laws make it out to be. For example, a number of test cases are now pending in state and federal courts throughout the country that might result in removal of the drug from its usual classification as a narcotic, along with heroin and other opiates, and in a lowering of penalties for its private, recreational use.

Many people who try cocaine in the United States must wonder why it is so popular. It is a very expensive drug, often selling for as much as $100 a gram, or $2000 an ounce. (The legal retail price in the pharmaceutical trade is $25 an ounce.) Usually it comes as a crystalline powder in various shades of white. Some people shoot it intravenously like heroin, but the vast majority of users snort it. When snuffed up the nose, it produces very quickly a strong sensation of numbness in the nasal passages and throat. Often, American black-market cocaine does little else. It is curious that people pay so much money to have their noses numbed.

The trouble is that most cocaine is highly adulterated before it reaches the individual consumer, usually with inert salts and sugars, sometimes with caffeine and amphetamines, and often with procaine and other synthetic local anesthetics that mimic the numbing action of the real stuff. Real cocaine, in addition to its local effects, provides a warm glow of physical and mental well-being, a feeling of energy and clarity without much of the body stimulation of amphetamines or caffeine. But this feeling is subtle and may require learning to perceive. Even with good cocaine, first-time users may not notice that they are high.

What cocaine seems to have going for it mostly is a powerful mystique. It is the rich man's drug, the drug of exotic decadence, a magic tool to prolong and intensify sexual experience. Moreover, the ritual of huddling together to snort precious grains of a forbidden delicacy has a certain romantic charm.

Until recently it was much easier to come across good cocaine in South America than in North America. I tried it perhaps a half-dozen times in the United States without ever feeling much beyond my nose and throat. Then, one afternoon in Cali, Colombia, at the apartment of some American dealers and musicians who loved cocaine, I complained that I had never really felt high from it. "Wait till you try this," one of them promised, chopping up the crystals with a razor blade and arranging them in thin lines on a mirror to be snorted through a rolled-up 100-peso note. I inhaled one line in each nostril, got the usual sensations, and then, unexpectedly, a strong feeling of strength and health that seemed to flow through my lungs into my chest and whole body. My mind became alert, calm, and clear. I remained in that agreeable state for an hour or so, after which I felt tired.

But that was in 1972. Today, much Colombian cocaine is as bad as most American, a logical result of so many Northerners coming down to score. My friend Jimmy, who knows his coke and has spent a lot of time in places where it is sold, tells me the quality of stuff on the Bogotá market has so declined in the past year that he is seldom tempted to buy anymore. "I've even seen it cut with borax," he says.

"These gringos come down here from New York and L.A. and think all they have to do is buy the first blow they see on the street, and it'll be better than anything they can get up there. The Colombians have learned they can sell just about anything and get away with it."

One thing I have noticed about the many gringos who come to South America to buy and use cocaine is that very few of them have any knowledge or experience of the plant that provides the drug they enjoy. That seems to be true, also, of the South Americans who use and traffic in cocaine. Yet the coca plant — "Mama Coca" to the early Spanish conquerors — has been, and is, an honored presence in the everyday lives of millions of native peoples of the New World. Its therapeutic values so impressed Europeans that they carried its use enthusiastically from the high Andes to their own continent. Only in this century has coca fallen into disuse among Europeans and Americans. Yet there has been increasing use of cocaine, the so-called active principle of the coca leaf. In my travels in South America I have made observations that point up distinct contrasts in the effects of coca and cocaine and that suggest all of us might benefit by paying more attention to the living shrub whose leaves were sacred to the Incas.

*

The coca shrub, *Erythroxylum coca*, is widely cultivated in eastern Peru and Bolivia, its probable area of origin. It grows there in the lush green valleys of the eastern slopes of the Andes, a region known as the *montaña*, at altitudes of up to 5000 feet. It is also cultivated, though less extensively, in northern Chile and Argentina, Ecuador, Colombia, throughout the Amazon basin, and in parts of the Old World, principally Java and Ceylon.

I first saw living coca while traveling by car in Bolivia in 1965. Steep hillsides were planted with the neat shrubs, most of them about three feet tall. In La Paz, the Bolivian capital, whole sections of the open Indian markets were given over to coca vendors. In these markets, rows of Indian women sat in identical postures, each before a mountain of dried coca leaves on a blanket. Each woman had a balance and a supply of large plastic bags, and for about twenty-five cents one could buy a great bagful of coca. Also set out on the blanket were dark gray, molded shapes of highly alkaline substances that must be used with the leaves. The alkaloids of coca are not released from the leaf except in alkaline solution. Indians in different parts of South America have devised different ways of alkalinizing their saliva.

In some places quicklime is used; in òthers, powdered sea-shells rich in lime, or the ashes of various plants. In Bolivia, most commonly, stalks of the quinoa plant, a local grain, are burned to ashes, mixed to a paste with water, then molded into shapes and dried. Sometimes this material is called *lejía*, the Spanish word for "lye," and it must be used with care because it is highly caustic. The first time I bought coca in the La Paz market, the woman who sold it to me showed me how to put a handful of dried leaves into my mouth, moisten them into a wad, then bite off a tiny chunk of lejía and mix it thoroughly with the wet leaves to avoid having it come into direct contact with my tongue. (I still got a few minor burns before mastering the technique.) The alkaliniz-ing substances differ in strength and flavor from region to region. In parts of Colombia, coca-chewing Indians carry small gourds of white powder (called simply *cal*, "lime"), which they spread on their quid of wet leaves with a stick. At times I have found it easier to use pinches of ordinary baking soda than the more powerful types of Indian "lye."

The flavor of coca is quite delicious, especially mixed with a bit of cal, lejía, or baking soda, all of which add a nice salt-iness. Most plants that contain alkaloids are bitter, and many leaves contain astringent tannins, but coca, especially when freshly dried, has a pleasing taste that most people like right from the first. In chewing coca, the idea is to build up a chaw of leaves about the size of a walnut and to main-tain that between the cheek and gums, letting the juices trickle down the throat. The leaves are not swallowed. After forty-five minutes or so, all the active material is extracted, and one can spit out the remains.

During the time that I stayed in La Paz it was very cold in the mornings. The lack of hot water where I was living made it an ordeal to get out of bed. I found that a morning chew of coca made it easier to start the day. I had never tried co-caine then and had no particular expectations of the leaves except that I had read a number of testimonials about them. I enjoyed the taste and the novel sensation of numbness in the mouth and throat, but I was disappointed that I did not feel high. At that time I did not realize that the high of coca is subtle, that it requires learning to appreciate, and that set and setting play a great role in shaping it.

I brought a bag of coca leaves and a bar of lejía back to the States from that trip and kept them around as curiosities. I remember that during my second-year pharmacology course in medical school, I shared them with several of my classmates and showed them how to chew. All of us experienced anesthesia in the mouth and liked chewing the leaves, but, again, none of us noticed that we were high. Thereafter, I lost interest in my bag of leaves and eventually threw them out.

I did not come across coca again until a number of years later, in the Colombian state of Cauca. Cauca is a mountainous region of southwest Colombia, and many of the Indians who live there are *coqueros*. But in Colombia, unlike Bolivia, coca is technically illegal. The leaves are not sold publicly except in small quantities by vendors of herbal medicines. In Popayán, the state capital, one can buy cocaine with ease, because the city is on the Pan American Highway. Much of the cocaine extracted in illicit laboratories in the Andes makes its way through Popayán en route to Bogotá and points north. But to get coca leaves in Cauca one must go to the hinterlands where Indians raise the shrub for their own use.

On one of my visits to Cauca I got some leaves from friends and chewed them with a bit of cal. That time I noticed the high. The experience left me eager to find out how to use the plant for best effect. Soon after, I met some Americans who were living in a remote valley, several hours hike over difficult terrain from the nearest village. They told me that coca made it possible for them to hike back and forth when they needed supplies.

Chewing coca to hike in the mountains is one of the most traditional uses of the leaves. Ancient Inca runners relied on coca to cover great distances in the high *sierra*, and their modern descendants still measure the length of journeys in terms of the *cocada* — the period of time that one chew of coca will sustain them. There are many reports of Indians being able to endure great physical hardship with little food as long as they have adequate supplies of coca. Here, for example, is a description from 1913 of the endurance of Indian porters near Popayán:

> After eating a simple breakfast of ground corn porridge, they would start with their heavy packs, weighing from 75 to more than 100 pounds, strapped to their backs. All day long they traveled at a rapid gait over steep mountain spurs and across mucky swamps at an altitude that to us, without any load whatever, was most exhausting. On these trips the Indians neither rested anywhere nor ate at noon, but sucked their wads of coca throughout the entire day. These Indians we found very pleasant, always cheerful, happy, and good-natured, in spite of the fact that their daily toil subjected them to the severest of hardships and the most frugal fare.*

Firsthand reports about Indian uses of coca usually emphasize that regular chewing of the leaf is consistent with good health, high social productivity, and long life. Moreover, much of the literature on coca talks about the therapeutic virtues of the leaf: Not only is it not harmful, it is said to provide nourishment for the body and to be useful in the treatment of many kinds of illnesses. On the other hand, some authorities who have no direct knowledge of Indians condemn coca chewing as a destructive habit.

To get more information on coca, I decided to visit some Indians who use it regularly. I also decided not to do that in the Andes, where cocaine has become so prominent. On the advice of a Colombian botanist friend, I flew from Bogotá to Mitú, the tiny administrative capital of the huge Territory of Vaupés, a stretch of the Amazon basin that borders on Brazil. Mitú's main street runs a few blocks, from the unpaved airstrip at one edge of town to the bank of the broad Río Vaupés at the other. In Mitú I found two Cubeo Indian boys who took me in a motored canoe up the Vaupés to the Río Cuduyarí, one of its tributaries, and then several hours up the Cuduyarí to a tiny village of Cubeos. I was assured that

* J. T. Lloyd, "The mamberos of Colombia," *Journal of the American Pharmaceutical Association* 2 (1913): 1244–51.

the Cubeos use coca constantly and are amenable to visits.

I arrived near midday on a brilliantly sunny Saturday in January 1974 in the midst of Amazonian "summer" — the dry, hot season when the rivers are low and clear and tranquil. It was a steep climb up the river bank to the village, a rectangular layout of ten thatched houses surrounded by forest. No one was outside; the sun was too intense. I had a note of introduction from the Catholic priest at Mitú to the schoolteacher of the village, but when I found his house, he was out fishing, and his wife spoke only a few words of Spanish. The boys explained who I was, and she indicated that I was welcome to wait. She offered me a large gourd of chicha, a natural, fermented beer made from *yuca* (tapioca root), and a large chunk of *casave*, the bread made from the same root. There was a gourd of fiery hot sauce, made from chili peppers and fish, for dipping the casave. As I ate and drank, the schoolteacher's wife went back to the cooking area and resumed her work of grating bitter yuca tubers — one step of the long process needed to remove their poisonous juices.

The house was spacious, dark, and unfurnished except for one table, a hammock, and a number of low, carved stools. An open fire burned low in one corner. I sat on one of the stools, looking out the door, relaxed by the rhythmic sound of grating. Outside, the sun was blazing. A few scruffy dogs lay in patches of shade, gnawing on fish bones. In the middle of the rectangular "plaza" of the village was an unfinished structure, the largest building of all, built of sturdy beams. I learned later it was to serve as a school and assembly house.

Before long the schoolteacher appeared with a mess of river fish. He was a short, intense man in a bathing suit and flowered shirt who spoke good Spanish. I addressed him as *maestro* and presented him with my note. He told me I was welcome in the village but would need the permission of the chief (*el capitán*) to stay. I told him of my interest in coca and he said there would be no problem in learning about it if I stayed. Then he told his wife to bring me another gourd of chicha, gave her the fish to cook, and played with his small children.

El capitán was an older man, very warm and thoughtful, who told me I could stay as long as I wanted. I assured him that I would pay for anything I needed and had brought with me sufficient gasoline for the return trip. (The boys who brought me had left for Mitú, but the village had a communal motor.) He showed me to one of the thatched houses, which was unoccupied, and said I could string up my hammock there. As I unpacked, he told me that it was a quiet time for him. Some of the people had gone off for several months to cut rubber, and only about thirty people were now living in the village. Besides, it was *puro verano* ("pure summer") — he gestured to the brilliant blue sky and puffy white clouds. That meant an abundance of fish, safe travel on the rivers, and a time of good health. I explained to the chief that I was interested in learning how his people cultivated plants, especially coca, and how they prepared them for use. He said he would be happy to take me to his own fields to show me.

Later in the day I spoke again with the teacher. He told me that coca, in the Cubeo language, is *patu*. Patu was the first Cubeo word I learned. As we talked about life in the village, a muffled thumping started up. The maestro stopped talking. "Let's go next door," he said. "They're preparing some patu now." We walked over to the next house. Its source was a tall wooden mortar, about eight inches in diameter and three feet high. The woman of the house was vigorously and rhythmically pounding a large wooden pestle. She spoke a few words to a young girl, who promptly served me a gourd of chicha. I was coming to like the tangy drink.

After a few minutes, the woman stopped her work and poured the contents of the mortar into a large gourd. What came out was a fine, bright green powder. She then reached into a pile of fluffy, gray ashes near the fire, scooped up a big handful, and added it to the powder, mixing with her hand until the color became a uniform, rich gray-green. Then she stopped as the maestro introduced me and explained that I was interested in coca.

"Would you like to try some?" the man of the house asked.

I said yes. He took a metal can off the shelf, opened it, and extracted a heaping spoon of the same gray-green powder, offering it to me.

"I don't know how to use it," I said. I had never seen coca prepared this way, although I had read that Amazonian Indians use powdered leaves mixed with ashes that supply the alkalinity. The man indicated that I should dump the whole spoonful into my mouth. I did so, and in the next instant fell on the floor choking.

"*¡Cuidado! Es peligroso,*" the maestro exclaimed. ("Careful! It's dangerous.") The powder was so fine that it created a miniature dust storm in my mouth. Inhaling before the dust settled was not advisable, it seemed. After a few difficult minutes, I recovered my ability to breathe and concentrated on masticating the coca powder into a workable mass. From time to time I breathed out green "smoke," but soon all the powder was moistened. I now had a large pasty lump in my mouth that I tucked to one side between cheek and teeth. Once the danger was over, I was able to concentrate on the excellent flavor of this Amazonian coca preparation. It was truly *sabroso*, as I told my hosts — a rich, toasted green taste, slightly smoky. Within a few minutes I felt a pleasant tingling and numbness spread through my mouth and down my throat. Soon after, I felt a warm, satisfying glow in my stomach. And then, little by little, my mood brightened, and I found myself exchanging warm smiles with the people in the house. They were all delighted that I enjoyed their patu.

I maintained the gob of paste in my mouth for about an hour, swallowing the juices that accumulated and occasionally licking off a dab and rolling it around my mouth. One advantage of this preparation is that it all dissolves eventually, leaving nothing behind to spit out. The good feeling it gave me lasted for some time after I had nothing more in my mouth; in fact, it never really ended but simply trailed off imperceptibly. By then the sun was setting, a lovely sight, and soon afterward a magnificently clear, starry sky was overhead.

The days I spent in the Cubeo village were long and

placid. Each morning people went off to tend their fields, the women were forever working yuca into casave or chicha, and at all hours of day and night men would go off in canoes to fish. The basic diet of the village was river fish grilled over open fires, casave, and chicha, with occasional ears of maize, dry-roasted. Hot chili peppers and limes were available and delicious pineapples as well. The other staple was *pupuña*, a starchy, orange-colored palm fruit* that was boiled, mashed, and fermented into another kind of chicha. The people looked well fed and in good health, although all of the children appeared to have gastrointestinal parasites. The most distressing environmental hardship was sandflies that abounded in great numbers and inflicted very irritating bites.

On the third day of my stay, el capitán took me with him in the morning to see his fields. I followed him along a trail through the forest for about half an hour until we came to a huge clearing planted with yuca of all sizes. Pineapples grew haphazardly among the yuca, along with a few pepper plants. I stumbled across giant fallen trees to keep up with the chief as he led me to his coca patch. "Patu," he said, gesturing to the little bushes. There were perhaps fifty plants, all about three feet tall, which looked as if they were being harvested continually. I rubbed some of the glossy-green oval leaves between my fingers.

"Every household grows its own coca?" I asked.

"Yes," the chief replied.

"Have the Cubeos always used coca?"

"Not always," he told me. "The old people say it was brought here a long time ago, but no one remembers how." He pointed to a large cecropia tree. *"Yarumo,"* he said.

"What do you use yarumo for?" I asked.

"For the ashes," he explained. Cecropias are members of the fig family and common denizens of the Amazon forest. They have giant, fanlike leaves.

"That's *yarumo blanco*," the chief went on, showing me that the underside of the leaves was silvery white. "It makes

---

* From the peach palm, *Bactris gasipaës*.

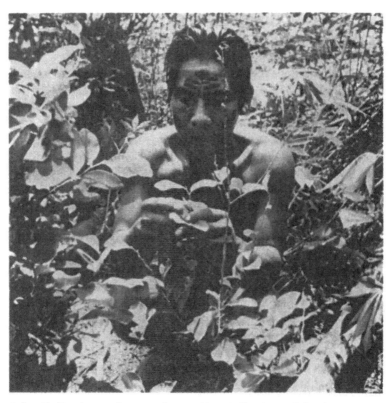

Cubeo Indian harvesting coca leaves, Vaupés Territory, Colombia. Amazonian coca, *Erythroxylum coca* variety *ipadú*, is a distinct form adapted to hot rain forests at low altitudes. Indians pick coca carefully by hand, leaving the terminal leaf on each branch. This practice encourages the plant to put forth new foliage. (Silvia Patiño)

the best ashes to mix with coca." I told him I hoped I would have a chance to prepare some coca with him from start to finish. He said we could do that soon.

That afternoon, nearly everyone in the village gathered in the shade of the unfinished school building to drink chicha, talk, and smoke the cigarettes I had brought as presents. Before long, several of the young men began playing reed flutes, and soon someone brought out the coca can and took it around, offering some to everyone. Most of the men helped themselves to generous amounts, but the adolescents and women generally declined. Coca was forbidden to women in the past; today, they may use it but usually do not. The green powder is almost exclusively a drug of adult men.

I took a spoonful and got it into a workable lump with only a few coughs. The impromptu party continued till sunset, interrupted only by a refreshing swim in the river. Great pots of chicha were served up throughout the afternoon, and the coca made another round. Chicha is mildly alcoholic, of course, but it does not seem possible to get really drunk on it. I discovered that I could drink from a gourd of chicha while maintaining the lump of coca in my cheek, letting it dissolve at its own rate.

My friend the schoolteacher became quite mellow after a number of gourds of chicha and began to tell me how proud the Cubeos were of their heritage as *indígenas*, natives of the Vaupés. Some of the men began dancing while playing their reed flutes, and in the fading light the rhythm of their fast steps and the curious melody put me into a trancelike state. I recalled that the Kogis of northern Colombia use coca to induce meditative states in religious ceremonies.

"Tomorrow, we'll go to cut trees." It was the chief speaking to me.

"Cut trees?" I asked.

"To make more fields," he explained. "We'll leave early."

"Early" meant just as the sun was coming up. The men of the village painted their faces with a dark red pigment and assembled at the house of one family, armed with machetes and axes. Then we all drank chicha, fortified ourselves with good doses of coca, and marched off into the forest. By now I had learned how to put the green powder into my mouth without difficulty. I found myself marching along in the column of Cubeos, swinging my machete, humming a tune, and feeling increasingly happy. The coca seemed stronger at this hour of the morning. Its warm glow spread from my stomach throughout my body. I felt a subtle vibrational energy in my muscles. My step became light, and there was nothing I wanted to do more than just what I was doing.

After a long, brisk walk we arrived at the area to be cleared and spread out to tackle the trees. The Indians were very protective of me and took great pains to keep me at a

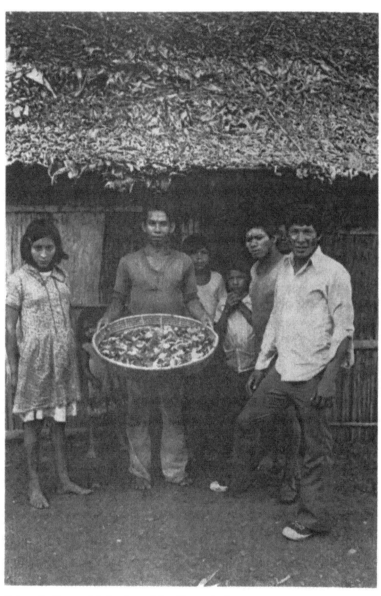

Cubeo Indians with basket of freshly picked coca. Amazonian coca has a tough, heavy leaf with a low cocaine content. The traditional preparation of it into a very fine powder mixed with ash makes it easier to consume as well as more powerful. (Steve Shouse)

distance when a giant tree was about to crash down. We worked for about three hours until a large section of forest had been cleared of trees and we were all tired, thirsty, and hot. The men explained that in a short while the area would be burned out, then eventually planted with yuca. We walked back to the village, where the women awaited us with chicha and casave, then went to the river to bathe. It had been a good morning's work.

The following day, the chief took me out with one of his young daughters to gather coca from his fields. We picked leaves from each plant, being careful not to remove the topmost. It took us about an hour to fill a large basket. The sun was so hot that I was glad when we finished our harvesting and started back. On the way we paused to collect a bunch of cecropia leaves to burn to ashes.

Back at the chief's house, the basket stuffed full of coca leaves was emptied into a large earthenware cooking pan, about four feet in diameter and eight inches deep. Made of baked river mud, it was usually used for cooking casave. The chief's wife placed the pan over an open fire, adding more wood to build up a good heat. Then, using her hands and a large paddle woven of reeds, she kept the leaves in constant motion, tossing and rolling them so that they would toast uniformly. She did this for about a half-hour until the leaves were crisp and dry, retaining their bright green color.

I put some of the toasted leaves in a plastic bag to take back to Bogotá. The rest were placed in one of the tall wooden mortars I had seen in use on the day of my arrival, and the chief and I and an old man who joined us took turns pounding them into powder. Meanwhile the cecropia leaves were placed over the fire to burn. When the coca had been reduced to a brilliant green powder, the chief examined some for fineness and then added ashes until the color darkened to his satisfaction. He next placed this mixture in a fine muslin sack and shook it vigorously inside a can; only the finest dust sifted through. When the flow of dust through the sack began to ebb, he poured the remaining powder back in the mortar — it was now bright green again — added

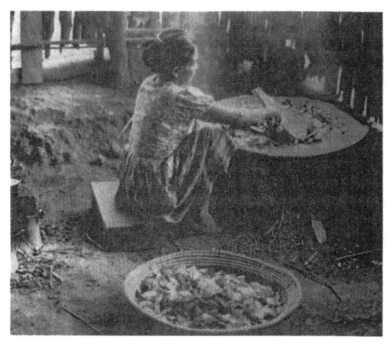

Cubeo woman toasting coca leaves. The fresh leaves are placed on a hot earthenware cooking slab over a wood fire and are tossed about with a woven paddle for ten or fifteen minutes until they are very crisp. This process gives them a distinctive smoky taste. (Silvia Patiño)

more ashes, and resumed pounding. We repeated this operation five times, helping ourselves to the finished product to make the work go faster. At the end of the fifth sifting, all that was left in the sack was some fiber. The can was full of gray-green patu, just the same as that in every household in the village. The experience of working with coca in this long and natural way, starting from the living plant, intensified my appreciation of the prepared material.

During the time that I lived with the Cubeos I saw coca used only at the start of communal work parties and at fiestas, when it was consumed in moderation, mainly by men, always accompanied by chicha and music. Although every house had a supply of prepared coca, I saw no one dip into the supplies except in the company of others for purposes of

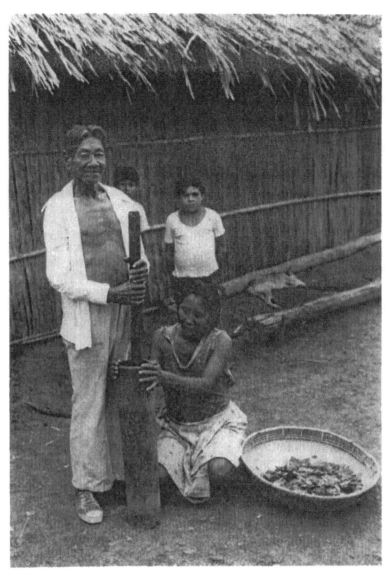

Cubeo couple pounding coca in a mortar. The toasted leaves go into this heavy wooden mortar, made from a hollowed hardwood log, and are pounded into a very fine powder with a stout wooden pestle. The initial pounding lasts about fifteen minutes and produces a thumping sound characteristic of Amazonian villages where Indians use coca. (Steve Shouse)

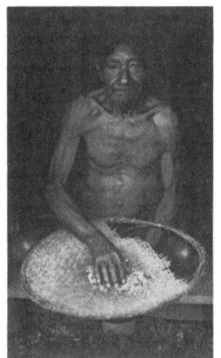

Left: Cubeo man sifting *Cecropia* ashes. Ashes of the leaves of a few species of *Cecropia* trees provide the alkali in Amazonian powdered coca. The huge dead leaves of these trees are gathered and burned. The ashes are then sifted and added to the pulverized coca. Initially, about an equal volume of ash is mixed with the powdered coca until the proper gray-green color results. If the mixture contains insufficient ash, its effect is weak. (Steve Shouse)

Right: Cubeo man sifting coca. In the final step of preparation, the coca-ash mixture is shaken through a cloth bag into a can. The stick in the bag keeps the mixture agitated. Only the finest dust comes through. When the flow slows down, the bag is emptied into the mortar, pounded again, mixed with more ash, and resifted. The material in the can is ready for use. After four or five cycles of pounding and sifting, only a small amount of fiber remains in the bag. (Silvia Patiño)

work or recreation. Young people rarely used it. I took coca
almost every day and each time found it tasty and plea-
santly stimulating. I developed no craving for it, no desire to
increase the dose, and no sense of becoming tolerant to the
effect. I saw no evidence among these Indians that coca use
was addictive or dependence-producing, nor that it was injurious to health. Some old men in the tribe had used coca all
their lives and still were satisfied with the occasional consumption of ordinary doses.

When I finally left the village to go back to Mitú and
thence to Bogotá, I carried with me my can of powder and
bag of toasted leaves. I was eager to tell people about the
virtues I sensed in this plant and to explore its possible uses
in modern medicine.

*

Cocaine is for horses, not for men;
They tell me it will kill me, but they won't say when.
Cocaine — run all 'round my brain.
                              — TRADITIONAL BLUES

In 1860, Albert Niemann of Göttingen, Germany, isolated
cocaine from coca leaves. Twenty-four years later, Karl Koller, a friend of Sigmund Freud, recognized its local-anes-
thetic properties. Although these discoveries were major
breakthroughs in modern pharmacology and medicine, the
appearance of cocaine in Europe and America had unfortunate repercussions that echo down to the present day. As
Richard Martin writes in his excellent paper, "The Role of
Coca in the History, Religion, and Medicine of South American Indians,"

. . . the discovery of cocaine had another less beneficial effect on
the reputation of the coca plant; for the occasional abuse of this
alkaloid, particularly among persons already addicted to opiates,
which was sensationalized by the press both in Europe and the
United States at the end of the 19th Century, created the errone-
ous fear that coca equalled opium in its perniciousness and its
deleterious effect on physical and mental health. In the space of

twenty or thirty years, coca went from high praise by kings, popes, artists, and doctors as the most beneficial stimulant tonic known to man to vigorous condemnation as a dangerous addictive narcotic. The effect of this prejudice and the subsequent legal ban on coca leaves in Europe and the United States was to halt experimentation with and use of coca leaves by doctors; only specialized uses of cocaine in anesthesia were regarded as acceptable. Even more serious, however, is the fact that confusion about the effects of crude coca leaves and those of cocaine has caused many people to regard the chewing of coca leaves as practiced by the Indians of South America as merely an addictive vice, with the lamentable result that coca is now being suppressed even in areas where the Indians have relied on its stimulating and medicinal properties for thousands of years, and where it has formed a significant part of their religious and cultural heritage.*

Under U.S. law, cocaine is classified as a narcotic along with opium and its derivatives. There is no medical justification for this classification. Narcotics are drugs that induce stupor; cocaine is a stimulant. Moreover, regular use of cocaine does not lead to one of the classic phenomena of narcotic addiction, a withdrawal syndrome upon the sudden discontinuance of use. For this reason, pharmacologists say that cocaine does not cause physical dependence. Nor is there any hard evidence that cocaine causes general physical damage to the body, though it has been accused over the years of harming the nervous system in all sorts of ways.

In one person who was shooting cocaine in Colombia, I saw a tendency toward orally aggressive and hostile behavior during the acute effect of the drug. Some snorters experience anxiety reactions to high doses. But I have never seen cocaine produce real aggression, violence, or psychosis. Among the hundreds of cocaine users I have known, I have only seen the drug induce good moods. Typical users enjoy talking and listening to music while high.

It would appear that many of the beliefs about cocaine

---

* Richard Martin, "The Role of Coca," *Economic Botany* 24, No. 4 (1970): 422–23.

that have led to current law enforcement practices are unfounded and have their origin in the hysterical fears of past days when cocaine was judged guilty by association, particularly with opiate addicts. For example, in sustaining unusually harsh sentences for two young men convicted of distributing small amounts of cocaine, a federal judge in Massachusetts in 1974 justified his action by citing this paragraph from the 1970 Working Papers of the National Commission on Reform of the Federal Criminal Laws (p. 1085):

> Cocaine is a powerful stimulant. While it does not cause physical dependence, a very strong psychological dependence upon cocaine can be developed. In the United States it is usually taken by heroin addicts in combination with heroin — as a "speedball," but occasionally people take it alone. It is not more often used alone because it may produce acute anxiety and may precipitate psychotic episodes . . . It should be classified as a dangerous drug because it may precipitate acute anxiety and psychotic episodes, and there is a strong possibility that such episodes may involve aggressive or violent behavior.

These ideas are terribly inaccurate. The vast majority of American cocaine users take the drug rarely or occasionally, only by nasal route, and in diluted form. They do not also use opiates and do not become aggressive, violent, or psychotic. Presumably, as more and more middle-class, "respectable" citizens try cocaine, the old attitudes will slowly change.

In defending cocaine against the attacks of misinformed persons, I do not mean to suggest that the drug is innocuous or beneficial. I see two main problems with it.

The first is simply that cocaine does not miraculously bestow energy on the body. It merely releases energy already stored chemically in certain parts of the nervous system. Consequently, when the immediate effect of the drug wears off, one feels "down" — less energetic than normal. The down following the high of cocaine is very noticeable and discourages some people from using the drug more than a few times. "I really like the way I feel after I snort it," one user told me, "but I can't handle the feeling two hours later."

This pattern in the effects of cocaine makes it a perfect object for the behavior of dependent persons because the simplest way to get out of the down phase is to take another snort. In the United States cocaine is too expensive for most people to use with any regularity, but whenever I have been around people who have access to large amounts, I have seen how easy it is to get into using it all the time. Once, in Ecuador, I stayed briefly with a group of Americans who used a lot of a crude form of cocaine known as *pasta*, which is the water-insoluble free alkaloid together with many impurities. Pasta comes as tan or brown lumps and is smoked in mixtures of tobacco or marijuana. In the illicit trade it is the next-to-last step in the manufacturing process. When reacted with hydrochloric acid, pasta forms the white, soluble hydrochloride salt of cocaine that is the usual commercial form. When I smoked pasta I found it powerfully stimulating but very short-acting, with an even more powerful depressant phase. I commented on this to my hosts, and one woman replied, "Yes, it certainly has a hook in it, doesn't it?" She then lit another pipe.

The second problem with cocaine appears when one bites the hook and uses more of the drug to relieve the depression. Tolerance to the high of cocaine develops rapidly, so that a second dose gives a less intense effect that lasts a shorter time. Users who have access to large amounts of cocaine can find themselves, very quickly, using it all the time and not doing much else. I saw a number of Americans in Colombia who spent most of their waking hours in unfurnished rooms snorting coke to the exclusion of most other activities. But I must repeat that this pattern seldom occurs in the United States, where cocaine is so expensive and so highly adulterated.

Besides these two pharmacological problems of post-stimulatory depression and rapid subjective tolerance, there are several other drawbacks to cocaine. For one thing, it is irritating to the membranes of the upper respiratory tract. On two occasions, within twelve hours of snorting moderate doses of cocaine, I have come down with colds that began as sore throats, probably triggered by the irritation. Possibly some of this effect is due to adulterants or contaminants of black-market cocaine. (More than once I have come across samples of Colombian coke that reeked of hydrochloric acid. Doubtless, the crystals were rushed into packages without proper washing.) But cocaine on its own powerfully constricts small blood vessels in the nasal membranes. For this reason it clears the nasal passages. Over a long time, snorting cocaine certainly leads to local weakening of tissue by interference with blood supply. Rare individuals who use it in great excess may even develop perforations of the nasal septum.

Furthermore, I do not believe we are meant to put powerful drugs into our systems by the nasal route. When cocaine is snuffed, it rapidly and directly enters the bloodstream. The "rush" of stimulation that some users like is largely due to the rapid increase of concentration of drug in the blood that follows this method of administration. Snorting is only one step down from intravenous injection. Like shooting, it by-passes many of the mechanisms our bodies have for protecting us from the adverse effects of foreign substances. When we put a drug in our stomach, we allow the body to decide how fast to admit it to the bloodstream and give the liver and kidneys time to work at metabolizing and eliminating it.

It is hard to convince persons who like cocaine that they would be better off eating the drug than snorting it. Taken by mouth, cocaine is less potent — that is, one needs a bigger dose. Therefore, eating cocaine is economically unfeasible for most users. Also, oral cocaine does not provide as fast a rush. But neither does it cause the same degree of post-stimulatory depression nor such rapidly developing subjective tolerance.

I must cite a final and troublesome problem with cocaine: the difficulty of leaving it alone. It is terribly hard for people who like the stimulation of cocaine to let the drug sit around unused. The white powder seems to exert a strong attraction even if it is kept out of sight.

In the preceding chapter's analogy between white sugar and heroin, I stated my belief that the refining of natural substances into white powders is dangerous because the powders are hard to control. More natural forms of reinforcing substances appear to carry certain messages that dictate appropriate use. These messages may be carried in part by the associate substances that occur in plants. Panela has many things in it besides sucrose, the sweet essence, and these other things convey strange tastes that keep us from consuming more than the body needs. In the same way, opium contains many compounds other than morphine, its active essence, and it is likely that these associate substances provide a kind of pharmacological insulation that protects users from the naked, hard-to-control effect of morphine.

It should come as no surprise to learn that cocaine is but one of a number of physiologically active chemicals in the coca leaf. To date, some fourteen alkaloids have been isolated from the plant. Pharmacologists have burdened us with the notion that drug plants must owe their properties to single "active principles" that can be isolated, synthesized, studied, and administered in pure form. This notion may be helpful to pharmacologists in making their experiments simpler, but it is harmful to the rest of us because it leads us away from natural green medicines in the direction of white powders with far higher potentials for abuse.

Richard Martin states the problem well:

> . . . the effects of the coca leaf often have been presumed to be embodied in the alkaloid cocaine, albeit in a more potent form, with the result that the majority of the physiological research for the last fifty years has been performed solely with cocaine and not with other preparations of coca leaves. However, many physicians have emphasized that the effects of these two are not identical, and particularly that the therapeutic qualities of coca are not represented completely in the active principle cocaine. An important consideration in this regard is that active principles and particularly alkaloids can exert quite different effects when administered as they are naturally combined in the plant than when administered in pure form. Very little is known about the physiological activity of the associate alkaloids of the coca plant,

and still less about their effects in combination. The necessity of looking into the possible importance of these other compounds is emphasized by the fact that an Indian will frequently reject the bitter coca leaves with the highest percentage of cocaine in favor of the sweeter leaves which are richer in the more aromatic alkaloids.*

Cocaine today has little use in medicine. Doctors sometimes use it as a topical anesthetic in the eye, nose, mouth, and throat. For local anesthesia by injection, it has been replaced by a number of synthetic "-caine" drugs that have no effects on consciousness. In isolating cocaine from coca and equating the effects of the leaf and alkaloid, European and American scientists not only gave the world a troublesome chemical but also deprived themselves of the benefits of a most useful plant. In so doing, they dishonored the spirit of Mama Coca. The sad results may well be her just retribution.

*

According to Indian tradition, coca was a gift from heaven to better the lives of people on earth. Over the years, South American Indians have found the leaf beneficial in numerous ways. Aside from its ability to clear the mind, elevate mood, and make energy available, it appears to exert good influences on many physical functions. For example, it tones and strengthens the entire digestive tract, possibly regulating carbohydrate metabolism and enhancing the assimilation of nutrients. A hot-water infusion of coca, sweetened with a little panela, called *agua de coca*, is a common remedy for indigestion and stomachache that is used even by non-Indians in parts of South America.

Coca appears to maintain teeth and gums in a good state of health, and it keeps teeth white (although use of caustic alkalies with the leaves may irritate oral membranes). The leaf is rich in vitamins and minerals, particularly A, riboflavin, E, and calcium. An average daily dose of coca (one to

* Martin, "The Role of Coca," p. 436.

two ounces) supplies an Indian of the high sierra with much of his daily vitamin and mineral requirement. Coca appears to have a beneficial influence on respiration and to effect rapid cures of mild altitude sickness. It is said to rid the blood of toxic metabolites and alleviate arthritis. Indians say that regular use of coca promotes longevity as well.

When European doctors carried coca back to their continent, they were able to confirm many of the therapeutic powers attributed to it and prescribed it widely to patients. Proprietary tonics based on coca became extremely popular. Our own Coca-Cola is an emasculated descendant of one of these nineteenth-century preparations.

My personal experiences with coca leave me convinced that the leaf is pleasant to consume and moderately stimulating in a useful way. It does not appear to be associated with dependent behavior or to provoke development of tolerance. It can be left alone if one chooses.

By contrast, cocaine is much less pleasant to consume, easily becomes associated with dependent behavior, is not very useful, and is very hard to leave alone. Yet in our society a great many people are using cocaine. Hardly anyone has seen a coca leaf. How have we managed to create such a situation?

Drug abuse is much more than the use of illegal and disapproved drugs by some members of society. It is the whole mentality that leads a society to make available to its citizens worse drugs rather than better ones, and many of us contribute to that mentality. The pharmacologist who teaches that coca and cocaine are equivalent, the physician who esteems synthetic white powders above natural green preparations, the judge who believes that cocaine is used mainly in combination with heroin are all as much responsible for unwise use of drugs as the user who takes cocaine in excess.

Throughout all of the argument as to why people use illegal drugs, we sometimes fail to notice the obvious: that people tend to use whatever is available. Over the past eighty years, everything we have done as a society to "protect" people from potentially harmful drugs has served to make worse preparations more and more available. The situation with cocaine is a paradigm of the process.

If a demand for a drug exists, it will be supplied. The demand for cocaine in our country is high, and black-market traffic in it will grow. There is no chance of curtailing the use of cocaine by trying to cut off the flow of it or by punishing users and sellers. There might be a chance of trying to interest users in coca and thereby encouraging them to shift their attention to something distinctly better.

On returning from the Amazon, I shared my coca with a number of cocaine users. All of them liked it and some said they would like to use it instead of cocaine. Of course, I told them a lot about the leaves in advance so that they chewed them with a good set. Set and setting are especially important in shaping reactions to natural drugs like coca.

Ignorance about coca is widespread. Not only have few cocaine users ever seen a coca leaf, many of them do not even know that coca exists. Some people who have heard of coca confuse it with cacao, the source of chocolate and cocoa. I have met almost no American physicians who are knowledgeable about coca.

I have often written that mental states triggered by drugs are latent in our own nervous systems and may be elicited by a variety of nonpharmacological methods. Yet I do not think it is reasonable to expect most people to be able to do without pharmacological aids. The use of drugs in our country is very great, and many of the legal ones, such as alcohol, tobacco, coffee, and tranquilizers, cause more social and medical trouble than some of the illegal ones. It is unrealistic to think we can make drugs go away, but we can teach people how to use them in better ways. One step in that kind of education would be to explain that natural drugs are less of a problem than isolated active principles and that certain natural drugs, like coca, are beneficial if used occasionally and with respect for their power.

The Indians I know who use coca respect their drug. They honor Mama Coca by treating her plant reverently, preparing it for use carefully, and guarding its power by saving it for occasions when they need it.

14

SOME NOTES ON *DATURA*

A *Datura* FLOWER opened in my garden last night: a great
showy bloom, white as moonlight, that perfumed the desert
air with its fragrance. The species in my garden is *D. meteloides*, also called *D. inoxia*, a common weed of Mexico and the
American Southwest. It is known here in Arizona as Sacred
Datura, sacred because of its long association with Native
American medicine, religion, and magic. Like all of its relatives in the genus (about twenty species in both Old and
New Worlds), and many of its more distant cousins in the
nightshade family, the Sacred Datura is strongly psychoactive. All parts of the plant are powerfully intoxicating, and
people have used it for thousands of years to induce significant, even violent, changes of consciousness.

Datura is not a nice drug. Although sometimes classified as
a hallucinogen, it should not be confused with the psychedelics. It is much more toxic than the psychedelics and tends
to produce delirium and disorientation. Moreover, *Datura*
keeps bad company. All over the world it is a drug of poison-
ers, criminals, and black magicians.

Despite its toxicity and bad reputation, *Datura* continues
to exert great fascination over young people. Drug crisis
centers in the American Midwest report increasing incidence
of acute intoxications by Jimsonweed (*Datura stramonium*)
among teenagers. I receive a surprising number of inquiries
about *Datura* from persons who want to try it. For example,
a man in California wrote me: "I have had no hallucinogenic
drugs. My work and pleasurable interests have taken me to

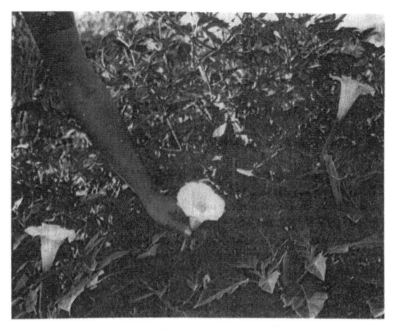

Sacred Datura, *Datura meteloides*, growing in a typical roadside habitat in Pima County, Arizona. The white blossoms open at dusk and close shortly after dawn. (Andrew Weil)

considerations of color and its characteristics. I am creative and visual and want to explore that part of my mind. I am interested in Jimsonweed. Can you recommend dosage, and do you think it wise of me to first use Jimsonweed, or should I use something else?"

To answer that question and those like it, I have collected some facts about these strange plants from personal experience and from reading.

Daturas, like other solanaceous (nightshade family) plants, such as Belladonna, Henbane, and Mandrake, owe their pharmacological properties to a group of chemicals called the tropane alkaloids. These drugs occur in all parts of the plants, including the flowers, with the highest concentrations in the seeds and leaves. The principal tropanes — hyoscyamine, atropine, and scopolamine — all block neurotransmission in the parasympathetic nervous system. The peripheral pharmacologic effects of these drugs are due to this parasympathetic blockade: rapid heart rate; dilated pupils; flushing, warmth, and dryness of the skin; dryness of the mouth; constipation; and difficulty in urinating and swallowing. In males, the tropanes also interfere with ejaculation. Toxic doses of these alkaloids produce fever, delirium, convulsions, and collapse. Death may occur in children, the elderly, the debilitated, and any persons unusually sensitive to the antiparasympathetic effects.

Some eaters of *Datura* experience nothing but physical toxicity. I once ate Jimsonweed seeds and had the following symptoms for forty-eight hours: a painfully dry mouth and throat, unrelieved by any amount of water; pupils so widely dilated that I had to remain indoors in a dim room; inability to focus my eyes at close range (a consequence of paralysis of the ocular muscles of accommodation); feverishness and restlessness; difficulty in initiating urination. Except for the restlessness and inability to concentrate, I had no particular psychoactive effects.

In clinical medicine, atropine and its chemical analogues are used as gastrointestinal antispasmodics, especially in cases of peptic ulcer and diarrhea. Atropine is also commonly injected subcutaneously in preoperative patients to dry secretions in the upper respiratory tract in order to facilitate intubation of the trachea and administration of anesthetic gases.

Atropine and hyoscyamine produce significant peripheral effects in ordinary doses but few changes in central nervous system functioning except near the toxic dose range. Scopolamine, on the other hand, commonly induces excitement, hallucinations, and delirium in subtoxic doses. Hence, scopolamine is the principal psychoactive component in *Datura* and other solanaceous hallucinogens.

During much of the twentieth century, scopolamine enjoyed great popularity in obstetrical medicine in the United States. Under the name "twilight sleep," it was injected into millions of women in labor to make them amnesic for the experience of childbirth. Obstetricians thought of it as a drug that simply erased memory for a few hours, and women who did not want to know anything of their labor and delivery liked it in retrospect. In 1966, as a third-year medical student in Boston, I took several weeks' training in obstetrics at a prestigious teaching hospital where scopolamine was still in vogue, and I watched many women under its effects. Anyone interested in altered states of consciousness who sees such cases will realize quickly that scopolamine is not simply an amnesic drug. Rather, it causes extreme confusion and disorientation, especially to people in pain. Women in labor who are "scoped" often appear agitated, hostile, even deranged. They writhe, scream, curse, and groan — hardly behavior that justifies the seductive term "twilight sleep."

In my opinion, the amnesia that follows this traumatic experience is not a direct effect of scopolamine but an inability to maintain continuity of awareness through such violent distortions of consciousness. The "scoped" woman is not unconscious. Her ordinary waking consciousness is fragmented. What comes through is primitive material from deep layers of the mind, strongly colored by pain and fear. People well versed in the repertory of altered states, who are familiar with deep meditations and trances or have trained themselves in the art of conscious dreaming, might be able to retain awareness through a scopolamine-induced delirium and not be amnesic afterward. People unfamiliar with such states do not have a chance.

Far from simply erasing a portion of experience, scopolamine releases such intense energies from the unconscious that the experience is later repressed and becomes inaccessible in the ordinary waking state. I have no doubt that women who deliver under scopolamine would recall their experiences under hypnosis and find them intensely unpleasant. Neither do I doubt that scopolamine strongly influences the birth experience of the baby, if only because of the state of the mother. Back in 1966, when obstetricians did not think of babies as conscious entities, no one considered this aspect of procedures in childbirth. Today, women are more interested in participating consciously in childbirth, and some obstetricians think about the impact of what they do on the newborn. Scopolamine, not unhappily, has passed out of general use.

In labor, scopolamine delirium is violent and terrifying, but it is hard to know whether this quality is inherent in the drug or is a result of the drug in a particular situation. Labor itself produces significant excitement and changes in consciousness. Also, obstetricians always gave scopolamine in combination with opiates and other psychoactive drugs.

If we look over accounts of *Datura* intoxication far from clinical settings, we find the same thing: It is a violent experience, often characterized by terrifying hallucinations and delusions, and frequently followed by some degree of amnesia. Here, for example, is a typical *Datura* experience, recounted by a young man who drank a tea of *toloache* (the Mexican name for *D. meteloides*) on the Pacific coast of Baja California, where he had gone to surf:

> Jim and I were in Mexico and didn't have any more pot, but we did have some *toloache* that we found. We decided to make some tea and boiled the leaves and stems. I drank about three-quarters of a cup. About ten minutes later I started to feel high. Then we went to eat lunch at the house of Tacho, the Mexican woodcutter we were staying with. I did not eat much because I was feeling so stoned. Then Jim and I left the house and went separate ways.
>
> I do not remember what happened after that until I found myself sitting on the beach. It was very rocky where I was, and I was looking at a small rock formation about fifty yards out. The tide was high, and waves were breaking over one end of this little rock island. I was just sitting on the rocks on the shore. Then I looked to my left and saw two big creatures, about the size of large gorillas, with human features. Their skins looked burned and were covered with boils. They weren't wearing any clothes and had boils all over their bodies. I stared at them, and one of them mumbled something. Then I turned away and looked at the ocean and saw people standing on the rock island in the water. There was a woman and several children. The waves were getting bigger, and, as I watched, they washed the woman and two children into the water. I stood up, I think, to get ready to go in the water to help, but just then a small boat, about nine feet, ap-

peared between me and the island. There were two men in it, and they went to help one little girl who was drowning. As they were pulling her in, a wave crashed over the rocks and tumbled the boat over. After the wave passed, I did not see the boat or any of the people.

When I looked again, I saw Tacho with the woman and two children on the rock island. They were trying to hold on to a little reef connected to the island. The waves kept pounding them and dragging them back each time they struggled to get up. Tacho ended up with one little girl on his shoulders. I heard him say to her in English, "Hang on to my neck!" Then I saw Jim in the water. He was trying to help a little boy. Then a really big wave broke, and everybody went down. I took off my shirt and glanced at the creatures next to me. They were staring at me with one eye and keeping the other on the scene in the water. I said, "Should I go out?" but they just stared. I saw everybody go down under the water again, so I dove in to help. I swam to the rock island and climbed on top, but no one came up. I thought everyone had drowned. I watched for about ten minutes but saw no sign of anyone. Then I swam in to shore and got my shirt. Only one of the creatures was there; he had blankets wrapped around him.

I was very cold, so I ran to Tacho's house. Some other people were there, and I stammered out what happened. Then I saw Tacho talking to his wife in the kitchen. I didn't know what to think. I still thought Jim was dead. Then Jim came walking up to the house, and I gradually realized that none of it had happened. This all took about five hours, but I had no awareness of time, and there seem to be gaps in my memory. For two days afterward I could not read or see close up. Otherwise I was O.K.

Typical features in this account are the hallucinations of great vividness and organization, absence of insight into the relationship of the hallucinations to ordinary consensus reality or to the taking of the drug, and the fearful content of the experience. Why does *Datura* terrify? Perhaps scopolamine selectively stimulates areas of the brain that provoke fear when aroused. Perhaps the physical effects of tropane alkaloids condition the experience. Many persons who eat solanaceous drugs develop burning thirst, fever, and the sensation of the skin being on fire. These symptoms often lead to visions of hellfire. In fact, a common cause of death under the influence of *Datura* is drowning — the result of stumbling into deep bodies of water while disoriented, in an effort to quench the thirst and fever.

The ability of *Datura* to remove a person so completely from ordinary reality certainly accounts for its popularity among criminals. In India, where the purple-flowered *D. metel* is the principal species, bands of thugs, known as *dhatureas*, used the plant to stupefy their intended victims. (The botanical name *Datura* comes from *dhatura*, the Hindi name of the Indian species.) Use of *Datura* as a form of knockout drops has been common in many parts of the world. Here is an account from a seventeenth-century Spanish chronicler of a similar practice in Peru, using a *Datura* preparation called *chamico:* "Not long ago, it happened that a man whom I knew was walking with a companion who, having plans to rob my friend, gave him a *chamico* drink. This caused the man to lose his mind and to become so enraged that, naked for his shirt, he started to throw himself in the river. He was seized like a mad man and restrained. For two days, he remained in this condition, without regaining consciousness." *

In the New World, Indians have long known and used *Datura* for various purposes. Some tribes of eastern North America administered decoctions of Jimsonweed to young men in initiation ceremonies. The following comment on this custom by a Virginia historian is from the end of the seventeenth century. The Indians referred to are Algonquins, who gave Jimsonweed in the form of a drink called *wysoccan:*

> . . . the *Indians* . . . pretend that this violent method of taking away the Memory is to release the Youth from all the Childish impressions, and from that strong Partiality to persons and things, which is contracted before Reason comes to take place. They hope, by this proceeding, to root out all the prepossessions and unreasonable prejudices which are fixt in the minds of Chil-

---

* Bernabé Cobo, *Historia del Nuevo Mundo* (Seville: E. Rasco, 1653). Quoted in Hedwig Schleiffer, *Sacred Narcotic Plants of the New World Indians* (New York: Hafner Press, 1973), pp. 117–18.

dren. So that, when the Young men come to themselves again, their Reason may act freely without being bypass'd by the Cheats of Custom and Education.*

Jimsonweed was the first New World hallucinogen sampled by Europeans. Some of the first English explorers of Virginia ate the plant, possibly on the recommendation of local Indians, and lost their minds for a number of days. They named the plant Jamestown Weed; the present form is a corruption of that name.

Datura has also been used by shamans among North American Indians. Carlos Castaneda's account of the use of "Devil's Weed" (*D. meteloides*) by don Juan, a Yaqui sorcerer, parallels uses of other solanaceous intoxicants by Medieval European witches. Don Juan instructed Castaneda to anoint his body with an extract of *Datura* mixed with fat in order to have the experience of flying.

In South America, *Datura* is still very popular with Indian sorcerers. In certain regions of the Andes, Tree Daturas are common. These are small, gnarled trees, almost always covered with large, fragrant, trumpet-shaped flowers that come in shades of white, yellow, and red. Botanists now put them in a separate genus, *Brugmansia*, but they are still commonly known as Tree Daturas and have the same psychopharmacological properties as their low-growing relatives, scopolamine being the active principle of both. In parts of Colombia, Ecuador, and Peru a profusion of these strange and beautiful trees around a dwelling virtually advertises the residence of a witch doctor.

The center of diversity of the Tree Daturas and the presumed area of botanical origin is Ecuador. In the adjacent regions of Colombia, especially in the Valley of Sibundoy, use of these plants is very frequent among shamans of the Kamsa and Ingano tribes. They use different species for different purposes, and the purposes range from divination to determine the whereabouts of lost objects to healing ceremo-

* Robert Beverley, *The History and Present State of Virginia* (London: R. Parker, 1705). Quoted in Schleiffer, *Sacred Narcotic Plants*, pp. 131–32.

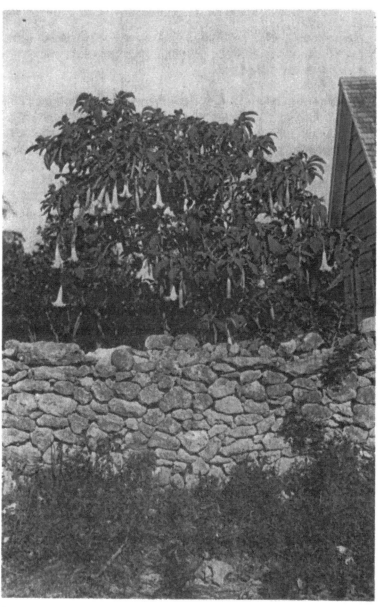

Tree Datura, *Brugmansia candida*, in the West Indies. These showy trees are native to Ecuador but are cultivated widely as ornamentals in the tropics of both hemispheres. (Courtesy Harvard Botanical Museum)

nies. Sibundoy Indians also add Tree Datura extracts to other hallucinogenic preparations like yagé.

The late Dr. Tommie Lockwood, who wrote a definitive monograph on the Tree Daturas, believed that these plants were well known to most Indian groups of western South America before the Spanish Conquest and were valued for both medicinal and psychotropic properties. Lockwood wrote: "It is sometimes difficult to separate these two properties in a shamanistic religion where there is a characteristic emphasis on malevolent magic and the supernatural as causes of illness."* Lockwood speculated that knowledge of the effects of Tree Daturas reached South America from Mexico by way of Indian immigrants from the North who knew *D. meteloides* and noticed the similarity of the flowers.

However, according to Michael Harner, an anthropologist and expert on the use of hallucinogens by New World Indians, *Datura* is not conducive to the subtle operations of the shaman:

> . . . the solanaceous hallucinogens are so powerful that it is essentially impossible for the user to control his mind and body sufficiently to perform ritual activity at the same time. In addition, the state of extended sleep following the period of initial excitation . . . together with the typical amnesia, make this hardly a convenient method for the daily practice of witchcraft. Furthermore, there is some ethnographic evidence that too frequent use of the solanaceous drugs can permanently derange the mind.
>
> I arrived at this particular insight about the problems of using solanaceous plants in shamanism and witchcraft during my field work among the Jívaro Indians of eastern Ecuador, who use both the solanaceous plant *Datura* and nonsolanaceous hallucinogens. They utilize the solanaceous plant in the vision quest, simply to encounter the supernatural, but do not use it in shamanism because it is "too strong" and prevents the shaman from being able to operate in both worlds simultaneously.†

*T. E. Lockwood, "A taxonomic revision of *Brugmansia* (Solanaceae)" (Ph.D. diss., Harvard University, 1973), p. 74.

†Michael Harner, *Hallucinogens and Shamanism* (London: Oxford University Press, 1973), p. 146.

To my mind, *Datura* is, indeed, too strong. Its physical toxicity is, at best, uncomfortable and, at worst, very dangerous. Its mental effects are unpredictable, often unpleasant, and always uncontrollable.

Once, in Colombia, I encountered a folk belief about *Datura* that appealed to me: going to sleep with a fragrant *Datura* blossom on your pillow is supposed to facilitate sleep and induce vivid dreams. (A similar idea has been recorded from Costa Rica.) I have followed this suggestion with blossoms of both Tree Daturas and the Sacred Datura of my garden in Tucson and found it agreeable. Inhaling the fragrance of the flowers is as close as I care to come to the psychoactivity of *Datura*. I enjoy being around these curious plants: They are fascinating and beautiful. But I prefer to admire and smell them rather than ingest them.

15

THE LOVE DRUG

MDA IS KNOWN as the love drug in the American subculture because of its reputation for producing loving feelings
in groups of people. The initials stand for 3,4-Methylene-
dioxy-amphetamine, and the drug is a straightforward derivative of amphetamine, first synthesized in Germany in
1910. Its effects on human beings are much more interesting
than simple stimulation. When I first encountered MDA in
1970, I took it a number of times and since then have observed its effects on a great many people.

The usual dose of MDA is 90 to 150 milligrams, taken
orally in a capsule. Its effects become apparent in twenty to
sixty minutes and persist for ten to twelve hours. People perceive the onset of these effects differently. Some experience
initial nausea. Some feel a warm glow spreading through
their bodies. Most people become aware of a sense of physical and mental well-being that intensifies gradually and
steadily. MDA commonly induces a state of profound relaxation and patience in which anxiety and defensiveness are
left far behind. "It is impossible to imagine anything being a
threat in that state," one user tells me.

Unlike most stimulants, MDA does not increase motor activity. In fact, it suppresses it in a remarkable way, so that
people can remain comfortable and content in one position
for long periods. This effect is most dramatic in people who
are heavily dependent on coffee and cigarettes, who are
always in motion of one sort or another. Under the influence
of MDA they, too, can be calm and motionless. Phar-

macologists call this the "antikinetic" action of the drug, but that is a negative way of describing something very positive. I prefer to call it a centering action.

The combined effects of relaxation and centering greatly facilitate certain kinds of physical activities, such as yoga, martial arts, and any disciplines requiring balance and maintenance of posture. For example, I can maintain a head-stand longer when I take MDA than normally. Although it is extremely pleasant just to lie still and enjoy a respite from nervous activity in this state, I have tried rock climbing and swimming after taking MDA and again find that my body works in a more coordinated, smoother fashion and that I can do more than usual. One novel experience, conferred temporarily by the drug, is the ability to interact with kinds of external stimulation that would ordinarily be painful and not get hurt. It may become possible to walk barefoot over sharp stones, for instance, and experience no discomfort or injury, apparently because the muscles are so free from im-posed tension that they can respond with precise coun-terpressure to the point of a stone. In this way, the skin feels no net force.

Such experiences confirm in a powerful way the sense of well-being. It feels as if nothing is threatening, and, in fact, things in the external world behave differently. This theme carries through to interpersonal relations. When people feel well, centered, unthreatened, and aware of their own strength and loveliness, they are able to drop many of the usual barriers that develop in groups. It is common in group MDA experiences for people to explore mutual touching and the pleasures of physical closeness. Participants may feel very loving toward one another, but the feelings are not ex-plicitly sexual because MDA tends to decrease the desire for orgasm. For many people the experience of enjoying physi-cal contact and feeling love with others in the absence of a specific hunger for sex is unique and welcome. (Some people do use MDA to heighten sexual experience.)

Other hungers and desires may also disappear in the MDA state. Habitual users of tobacco feel no need to smoke. Chain smokers of marijuana do not need their weed. Nail biters leave their fingers alone. Compulsive talkers become quiet. Compulsive eaters do not think about food. Moreover, this desireless condition feels supremely natural and valuable. Because MDA affects the senses minimally, everything appears as it does usually. There are no hallucinations, illusions, or distortions, simply a great aura of peace and calm. It is not possible to pretend, as it often is with hallucinatory drugs, that the experience is coming from without. Clearly, all of the important effects, including the ability to be free of anxiety and desire, are part of the human repertory, often unexpressed, to be sure, but there nonetheless.

The trouble with obtaining this state through the use of a drug is that it does not last. After five or six or eight hours, the old habits begin to creep back. Before long the experience of loving peace and desirelessness is in the past. The value of the drug is that it can show people that certain ways of being are possible and available; it gives no information about maintaining them.

I do not mean to paint a picture of MDA as a trouble-free panacea. Like all psychoactive drugs, its effects vary greatly with expectation and setting. People who take it in combination with alcohol and downers at wild parties with strangers are not likely to realize its potential. MDA also releases much energy stored in the nervous system, so that those who take it often feel tired and sluggish the next day. It should not be used unless one is in good physical shape with adequate energy reserves. For unknown reasons, it seems to be harder on women and may activate latent infections or problems in the female genitourinary tract. Women should take lower doses than men until they are sure the drug agrees with them and should avoid the drug altogether if their pelvic organs are ailing. Many people of both sexes report that the drug causes tension of the muscles of the jaw and face. In some individuals this effect becomes very annoying, progressing to involuntary grinding of the teeth. All of the adverse physical effects of the drug are dose-related. Whenever I have interviewed people who have had bad experiences with MDA, I have determined that they have taken excessive doses, been in poor settings, or taken other drugs masquerading as MDA.

In the right hands, MDA is quite safe. Out of hundreds of experiences with it that I have observed, I have seen only three anxiety reactions. The medical potential of the drug is great and quite unexplored. I have noted repeatedly that people under the influence of MDA, when feeling high, centered, and free of desire, are in a state of complete anergy — that is, they manifest no allergic reactions, even to allergens to which they have a lifelong sensitivity. Asthma disappears, hay fever disappears, cat allergies go away, and there are even no responses to mosquito bites. This effect is temporary and appears to be the analogue in the body of the mental experience of complete relaxation and lack of anxiety. It might be reproducible without the drug if we could learn to spend more time in that state. I can envision a training program in allergy control in which patients would go through ten sessions with decreasing doses of MDA in settings designed to maximize the centering effect and demonstrate the possibility of coexisting with allergens. By the tenth session the dose would be zero and patients would be doing it all on their own.

Unfortunately, the federal government, having declared MDA to be a drug with high abuse potential and no redeeming therapeutic value, has placed it in a category (Schedule I) that makes it unavailable to physicians and available to researchers only with difficulty. I know of no ongoing research with MDA in this country and consider this lack to be another result of unenlightened policies on substances that could be helpful to us.

16

READING THE WINDOWS
OF THE SOUL

IRIDOLOGY IS A SYSTEM of diagnosis of illness based on observation of the human iris. The iris is the colored part of the eye surrounding the pupil and is named for the rainbow goddess of the ancient Greeks, who, along with Hermes, carried messages from Olympus to earth. Although iridology has been around for over a hundred years, it remains an unorthodox science, not only unused by medical doctors but even unknown to most of them.

A delightful story about the origin of iridology is that the initial discovery was made by a ten-year-old boy, who, while playing with a pet owl, accidentally broke one of its legs. Soon after, he noticed the appearance of a dark stripe in the lower portion of the owl's iris on the same side of the body as the injury, a change that regressed as the leg healed. That event took place near Budapest, Hungary, and the boy, Ignatz von Peczely, grew up to become a medical doctor. Intrigued by his chance observation, he continued to look at irises, first of owls (easy) and then of people (harder), and eventually was able to establish a map correlating different areas of the body with specific parts of the iris. His first book on the subject was published in 1866. At about the same time, working independently, a Swedish homeopath named Nils Liljequist also discovered the principles of iris diagnosis. His writings were translated into English as a two-volume work, *Diagnosis from the Eye*, and it was Liljequist who first brought iridology to America.

Over the years, these early discoveries were refined by an unbroken line of practitioners following the precepts of von Peczely and Liljequist. Almost always these men adhered to systems other than allopathy, or orthodox Western medicine. For example, in the United States iridology is used mainly by chiropractors and naturopaths. Very few graduates of orthodox medical schools have even heard of it.

I came across iridology first by reading unorthodox literature on health, then by meeting someone who had had his irises read, and finally by tracking down a real, live iridologist who practices in Fairfax, California, north of San Francisco. Since then I have read a textbook of iridology, have looked at a number of irises, and have tried to put this new knowledge together with what I know from my orthodox medical training.

I am not able to say how accurate iris diagnosis is compared to the standard methods of physical examination and laboratory work. I do not have enough practical experience with iridology, and I am sure that skill with it, like skill with any diagnostic method, comes from practice alone. However, I am now well grounded in the theory of the system and can say something about that aspect of it.

The basic postulate of iridology is that all disease changes in the human body are reflected in the iris and can be read there by someone who knows the signs. To analyze this assumption, we can begin by noting that the iris is an organ made up of layers of different tissue, the bulk of which is muscle. There is a dark pigment layer deepest down, and a vascular layer that is more superficial, but most of the structures we see on looking at an iris are muscle fibers arranged circumferentially and radially around the pupil. The job of these muscles is to regulate the size of the pupil.

There is no question that our muscles live in intimate balance with our nervous systems. Muscles are literally nourished by nerves. If their nerve supplies are interrupted, muscle fibers wither away. The state of our nervous systems is revealed in the state of our muscles.

This simple idea, taken as truth by the most orthodox physiologists, ought to have important implications for medicine. For one thing, the nervous system regulates every aspect of bodily function. There is no cell in the body that is not under the direct influence of nerves, and through them, of consciousness. Therefore, we ought to be able to tell things about our bodies, our minds, and the relations between them by observing our muscles. That orthodox medicine has never pursued this line of inquiry is a consequence, I think, of two problems, one theoretical, one practical.

The theory (what there is of it) of orthodox medicine does not look at wholes like concepts of "vital energy" or mind-body interrelationships; instead, it concentrates on isolated mechanisms. The allopath sees muscles as an isolated system subject to certain specific diseases, like muscular dystrophy. He does not see them as an interface between mind and body in the whole organism. Wilhelm Reich, the great Freudian heretic who did pioneer work on the energy relationships between psyche and soma, insisted that psychological problems were manifested in physical ways, particularly by chronic muscular tension ("armoring"), and that they were susceptible to physical as well as psychological interventions. This insistence led to his ostracism from orthodox Freudian circles.

Reich has been dead twenty years, but his fame continues to grow, and his influence is now felt in many diverse systems of therapy. For example, Rolfing, an immensely popular technique of deep massage developed by Ida Rolf, is directly in the Reichian tradition. It is designed to restructure personality and body by working with the attachments of muscles to bones and by identifying and breaking up points of resistance in muscles that are believed to be physical correlates of painful experiences repressed into the unconscious. It seems to work for many people. As I have learned more about Rolfing and other types of massage, I am astonished that my medical education included not a single word on this subject. By contrast, many nonallopathic systems, such as classical Chinese medicine, place great emphasis on muscular manipulation — not simply as a method of alleviating symptoms in specific muscles but as a means of affecting general physical and mental processes.

Even systems that admit the theoretical possibility of using the muscles to understand the rest of the body face a practical difficulty: Muscles are manipulable but they are not directly observable. The tongue and anal sphincter are the only visible muscular organs other than the iris, and their fibers are hidden beneath coverings of epithelial tissue. For this reason the iris has a special claim for attention. It lies just beneath the cornea, the transparent window that admits light to the eye, and thus is the only muscle that can be observed directly. Moreover, as an integral part of the eye, the iris is even more special because the eye is a direct extension of the brain. Of all visible parts of the body, the iris alone affords a glimpse of our innermost workings. The term "window of the soul" seems very appropriate, as does the name Iris, the messenger of the gods.

It makes sense that all parts of the body are reflected in each part, that the state of the whole can be read in any part if one knows how to do it. Every orthodox physician knows that each cell contains the entire DNA code that has produced the whole body, and that every organ is linked to every other organ through the nervous system. I have seen a Mexican woman make sophisticated diagnoses by observing only hands. Acupuncturists can do the same by measuring pulses with great precision. If one could diagnose simply by looking at a visible structure, there would be less need to explore surgically or even to take blood from veins. Therefore, the possibility of seeing in the iris conditions in the rest of the body is worth considering.

The iridologist I met in California is Dr. Josh Carter, a young optometrist with a doctorate from the University of California. Dr. Carter came across the science of iris diagnosis when he was studying acupuncture at the North American College of Acupuncture in Vancouver, British Columbia. In his formal training in optometry he had never heard of it. Subsequently, he read a text called *The Science and Practice of Iridology,* by Bernard Jensen, a chiropractor and naturopath known as America's leading exponent of iridology. This text impressed Dr. Carter sufficiently that he went to visit Jensen, then in his sixties, at his Hidden Valley Health Ranch in Escondido, California, near San Diego. After watching Jensen work with patients, Carter decided to learn the method himself and now practices it routinely on patients who come to his Fairfax office. He is still learning traditional Chinese medicine and says he gets good consistency between iris diagnosis and the pulse diagnosis of the Chinese system.

Carter read my irises by examining them under a slit lamp, an instrument used to study the cornea in conventional medicine. It projects a narrow beam of light onto the surface of the eye and has magnifying lenses of different powers for close observation. After going over my irises, Carter guided me in the examination of a third person's eyes. I soon learned that it is much easier to look at blue eyes because their structure is much more visible; to examine brown eyes good illumination and some patience are necessary. But whether eyes are blue or brown has no significance in iridology.

What is significant is the density of muscle fibers in the iris. They can be tightly packed together like the fibers of silk cloth or the grain of a hard wood (oak), or they can be loosely meshed like the grain of a soft wood (pine) or the fibers of muslin or even burlap. Iridologists consider density to be an index of general vitality. The denser the fibers, the more inherent vital force a person has to withstand disease. Yet people whose irises show them to have high potential vital energy may, through poor life habits, be in worse shape than people with less energy who take good care of themselves.

After assessing the general density of the whole iris, an iridologist considers specific areas of lowered density. Any gap or hole in the iris is thought to say something about the state of a particular organ. The entire body is believed to be represented on the iris. In general, parts of the left side of the body, like the left arm and spleen, are represented on the left iris, while parts of the right side, like the right leg and liver, are represented on the right. The top of the body corre-

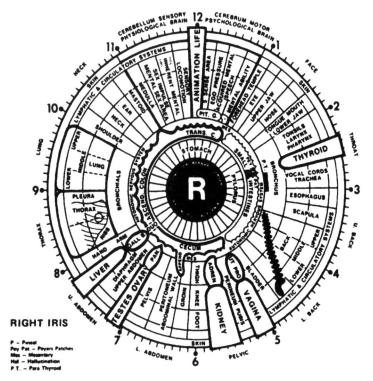

RIGHT IRIS

P – Pineal
Pey Pat – Peyers Patches
Mes – Mesentary
Hal – Hallucination
P.T. – Para Thyroid

Iridology chart developed by Dr. Bernard Jensen, D.C., Escondido, California, copyright © 1980 by Bernard Jensen, D.C.

sponds to the top of the iris, so that brain areas are represented on the arc between eleven o'clock and one o'clock on both irises, while indications about the legs and feet are found at six o'clock. The gastrointestinal tract, being most interior, is shown as a wreath around the pupil, and the skin, being most superficial, is mapped around the extreme periphery of the iris.

Since the time of von Peczely's owl, iris maps have been getting more and more specific. Reproduced here is the iridology chart developed by Bernard Jensen, in which left and right are reversed so as to correspond to the view of a patient facing the examiner. In his textbook, Jensen says he has tested this chart over years of practice and proved its value. He says also that when one finds a lesion in a particular

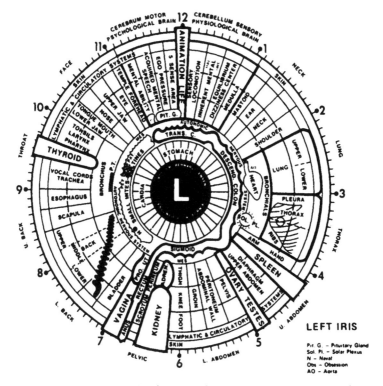

Pit. G. – Pituitary Gland
Sol. Pl. – Solar Plexus
N – Naval
Obs – Obsession
AO – Aorta

LEFT IRIS

organ area, one can tell whether the problem is acute, suba-
cute, or chronic by the appearance of the disrupted iris fibers, and, moreover, that healing is indicated by the filling
in of a gap with fine white fibers.

The possibility of representing the entire body on the iris
is suggested, no doubt, by the circular arrangement of the
muscles, for a circle denotes completeness. I do not have
enough evidence to say whether Jensen's highly detailed
map is more than fantasy. Dr. Carter did correctly spot a
man's upper back trouble merely by looking at his eyes
while I was present, and he showed me in a woman's eyes
the indications of a past tonsillectomy (two diamond-shaped
holes in the tonsil area). But he found a "prominent lesion"
in the upper lung region of my left iris (I can see it quite
clearly in a mirror), which a subsequent chest X ray shows
no evidence of. Might the wide gap in my left iris really be in
the adjacent shoulder and neck region? I have no known

trouble there either. So I remain skeptical about the mapping of the iris and the interpretation of "lesions" found there.

As practiced in this country, iridology is a philosophy of health as well as a diagnostic tool. Iridologists do not necessarily attempt to treat localized problems indicated by iris signs but rather to improve the overall well-being of the patient, particularly by the use of special diets and fasts and by the elimination of bad habits like smoking, overuse of drugs, and consumption of "unnatural" foods. If the patient follows a course of right living, his symptoms should regress. The iridologist ought to be able to follow the changes by observing the progress of healing signs in the eye. Jensen stresses the value of iris examination in preventive medicine and as a monitor on the effectiveness of treatment. "Iridology can be used," he writes, "in conjunction with any other form of analysis and diagnosis in helping a patient to a better state of health." In fact, he urges that it not be used as an isolated technique.

My brief acquaintance with iridology leaves me interested, skeptical, and eager for more information. Jensen writes: "I would advise the person who wants to see if there is anything to iridology not to come to any definite conclusions until he has spent at least three months with this form of analysis." I will try to look at irises from now on whenever I examine sick people. It is remarkable that orthodox medical men ignore the iris so completely in physical examinations. Even ophthalmologists have little to say about it, paying more attention to the cornea in front of it and the lens in back of it. The iris is a beautiful organ whose complex and delicate structure is easily observable. Doubtless, it contains much information about the general state of the body, possibly even information about specific problems. At the least, medical doctors should know that iridology exists, and some of them, I hope, will give it a try.

*

Although I have not done further work with iridology since meeting Dr. Carter, I continue to find people who practice it and believe in it. More than ever, I feel good diagnostic judgment involves a great deal of intuition coupled with observational talent and experience. I once met an old clinician who could pinpoint a patient's blood pressure just by watching the person in a hospital bed. He was almost always right but could not explain how he did it. I think he was a good observer with a good memory and a lot of experience who was willing to rely on intuition.

Medicine is much more of an art and much less of a science than many physicians care to admit. The science of diagnosis by taking readings and getting figures from laboratories may be less helpful than the art of diagnosis by shrewd observation. At least, the two should go together. Perhaps examination of the iris can serve as a convenient focus on which to project one's intuitions about a patient's problems.

Since my first brushes with unorthodox medicine, I have come across more and more of it. All sorts of practitioners are surfacing, and all sorts of people are turning to them for help. Patient dissatisfaction with regular doctors is at an all-time high, and the same three complaints are heard over and over: Modern medical methods are too expensive, too productive of adverse consequences, and not effective enough in treating the major killing and debilitating diseases.

Alternative medicine includes many practices, some of them sensible, others not. Systems of treatment are not right just because they are unorthodox; neither are they wrong automatically for that reason. Sorting through all the different systems takes time and patience. My hunch is that some of them have much to offer and might influence regular medicine in useful ways.

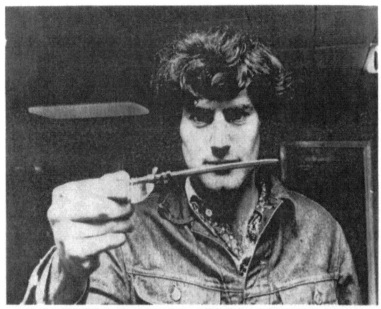
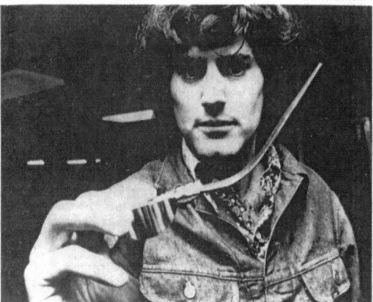
Uri Geller concentrates on a knife to make it bend. Moments later the knife is bent. (Topix Picture Service)

NOW YOU SEE IT, NOW YOU DON'T: THE MAGIC OF URI GELLER

Since the dawn of history various extraordinary phenomena have been recorded as happening amongst
human beings. Witnesses are not wanting in modern
times to attest to such events in societies living under
the full blaze of modern science. The vast mass of such
evidence is unreliable, coming as it does from ignorant,
superstitious, or fraudulent persons. In many instances
the so-called miracles are imitations. But what do they
imitate?

VIVEKANANDA, Raja Yoga

U RI (pronounced "Oorey," not "Yoorey") G ELLER, a
twenty-six-year-old Israeli, came to the United States in
1972 to demonstrate his abilities in telepathy and psychokinesis. Among other things, he claimed to be able to bend
or break metal objects just by concentrating on them and
even to cause things to dematerialize. Some of his powers
were vouched for by physicists at the Stanford Research Institute, a private think-tank in California that conducted
"controlled" tests of the "Geller effect" in the fall of 1972.
Uri was less interested in demonstrating his talent for scientists than for the general public. He appeared on national
television shows and performed before large audiences
across the country. Books and articles about him soon ap-

peared. In the process, Uri Geller became rich and famous and convinced many people that a new age of miracles was upon us.

I first saw Uri in early 1973 in Berkeley when he made one of his initial public appearances. The event was a meeting of the California Psychical Research Society and it took place in a school auditorium filled to capacity with people who had paid a moderate admission fee to see the Israeli Wonder. I sat about twelve rows back from the stage.

The program began with an introductory speech by Dr. Andrija Puharich, a physician and parapsychological investigator who discovered Uri Geller in Israel when Geller was working as a nightclub entertainer. Puharich explained to us that Uri was very tired because that day he had tried to demonstrate his powers before committees of Nobel Prize winners from Berkeley and Stanford Universities. He assured us that Uri had passed the rigidly controlled tests of the Stanford Research Institute with flying colors and that he was capable of amazing psychic feats. All we had to do was "be with" Uri — that is, give him our own mental energies.

Uri then came on stage. He was very charming, good-looking, and boyishly enthusiastic. He said that his day had been exhausting, expecially since he had not been able to produce any effects. The mental set of an audience is crucial to his performance, he explained. If people are "with" him, all sorts of things happen; but if people are not with him, nothing happens. As an example, he described his inability to do much of anything in the hostile editorial offices of *Time* magazine a short time before. But with the staff of an underground newspaper in the Bay Area he had been able to make pieces of silverware break and cause objects to dematerialize — vanish without a trace.

He said he requires other people's energies to work with; therefore, the bigger the audience the better. He likes to work with women because they are "more sensitive" to the powers he uses. He asked us to be patient with him: He would just talk for a while and not try to do anything until he felt like it.

He told us that he first became aware of telepathic abilities as a young child when he was able to guess his mother's hands at card games. When he was about seven, he noticed while sitting in class at school that the hands of his wristwatch would often jump forward or backward several hours. Eventually, he learned that these movements occurred when he willed them. Uri kept these powers to himself and as he grew older attached less importance to them. In his early twenties he became interested in them again, practiced at them, and finally decided he should use them to make his living. In mid-1970 he began appearing before small audiences. By the end of 1971 he was well known in Israel and had been seen by almost everyone there. It was at this time that he first met Puharich, who brought him to America.

Uri began his demonstrations by picking several female volunteers from the audience. He kept asking us not to be disappointed if nothing happened. "Just want something to happen, and maybe it will." He asked the first woman to write on a blackboard the name of a color. He did not look as she wrote *blue* and then erased it. Then he asked the whole audience to "think" the name of that color at him on the count of three. "And, please, no one whisper it," he cautioned. He counted to three. I thought *blue*. We repeated this three times. Uri shook his head. "I'm having some trouble," he said. "Once more. One, two, three . . ." There was a long pause. "O.K.," he said, "I'm going to take a chance. The color I get is blue." The audience applauded wildly. He held up his hands. "Wait. I must ask: Who over here" — he pointed to the right front section of seats — "was sending yellow?" A young man in that section gasped and raised his hand. "Please don't do that," Uri told him, "it really confuses me." The man apologized: "I couldn't help myself."

Uri was also successful at the next test: a foreign capital written on the board, erased, and then sent to him mentally by the whole audience. The capital was Prague; he got it with little difficulty. He also reproduced several figures drawn on the board.

"I'll tell you how I do this," he said. "I have in my mind a kind of screen, like a television screen, and when I receive something, whatever it is draws itself on that screen."

Uri then wanted to try some demonstrations of psychokinesis. He would first attempt to fix broken watches. "If anyone has a watch that is not running, as long as no parts are missing from inside, bring it up front, and I'll try to make it go." Apparently his talent at this operation was already well known because many people had brought their stopped watches with them. Uri fixed a watch by having a woman hold it in her hands and putting his hand over hers. Without touching the woman's hand, he passed his palm back and forth as if trying to direct some sort of energy. He asked his volunteer to let him know if she felt any sudden sensation of heat or tingling. She did. He opened her hands, took out the watch, and it was running. He repeated this demonstration with a number of other watches and got almost all of them to run. One was an antique pocket watch that had been stopped for years.

Elated by this success, he said he would try to bend some metal objects. Uri explained that objects to which people were emotionally attached were most suitable. Volunteers rushed forward with an assortment of rings, keys, and pins. He would not guarantee that he could do anything at all because he was so tired from his day of failures with the Nobel laureates. He tried bending several rings by putting them in the hands of volunteers and again passing his hands over theirs but got no results. After a number of attempts, he gave up. "No it just doesn't want to work tonight." The audience was only slightly disappointed; they had already seen so much.

Uri concluded his presentation by offering to take a group of volunteers on a blindfolded drive through Berkeley. That is, he would be securely blindfolded and would drive a car, using telepathic reception of the vision of the other passengers to navigate. There was no shortage of volunteers. I heard the next day that the ride had been successful and dramatic.

Uri Geller was now a real person to me, and a likable one at that. As for whether he really had the power of mind over matter, I could not say. I had not seen him fix the watches with my own eyes (I was sitting too far away), although I believed the testimony of those who had. I did not see him bend any metal. The telepathic experiments were entertaining, but they did not move me. I had seen stage magicians give similar or better performances using trickery. Blindfolded driving also does not really impress me — one can get very good at peeking through even the best-fastened blindfolds.

What I really wanted to see was a key bend or a ring break: That would decide the case. I should say at once that my prejudice is all on the side of believing such things possible. I have no doubt that telepathy exists. In fact, I think it is so common that we do it all the time without being aware of it or without attaching significance to it. Psychokinesis I have never seen, but I am willing to believe it can happen. Nor do I have to go through any mental gymnastics to rationalize its existence. The proposition that matter and energy are synonymous on some level is consistent with all of modern conceptions in physics. The proposition that human consciousness is a form of real energy seems to me self-evident. Why should consciousness not be able to affect the physical properties of objects?

I was perfectly willing to believe that Uri Geller could demonstrate that power. I also knew that seeing such a demonstration would not cause me to change my views of the world or of the mind. But it would be fun to see it.

*

By the time I saw Uri again, he was becoming famous in the United States. He had made convincing television appearances on the "Merv Griffin Show" and the "Jack Paar Show." On the latter he had caused a heavy metal spike to bend, to the astonishment of his host. Articles about him came out in many magazines, most of them favorable. Only *Time* accused him of being a fraud.

I was living in New York in June 1973, when Andrija Puharich invited me to a small gathering on the Upper West

Side. Uri would be meeting some people interested in making a feature film about him. When I arrived at the apartment, about ten people were present, among them Puharich and Geller. Uri had just flown in from California and was looking in good shape, although he said he was very tired. The company included a lighting director from a major television network with his wife; a young lawyer and his wife; a young woman psychic, also a protégée of Puharich; and Jascha Katz, one of two Israeli "promoters" who manage Uri's professional appearances.

Many of the people present had seen Uri perform well, and some of them had witnessed phenomena they considered miraculous. The lawyer showed me a ring Uri had bent for him and said the experience changed his life.

After some informal talk, we drifted into a small living room and sat down, hoping that Uri would feel up to trying out his powers. There were now about a dozen of us. Uri asked us to be patient and relax and rather than urge him to do things, just to talk with him. He began to tell us stories of his recent feats. He had "blown the mind" of an astrophysicist by causing his fork to bend while they were eating dinner together. The day before, on the plane in from California, he had "unconsciously" jammed the motion picture projector, causing film to spill out on the floor. "Things like that are always happening around me," he said. "Sometimes Andrija and I are eating in a restaurant and — *pop!* — a fork on the table is breaking just like that."

Someone asked Uri what he thought this power was. "I don't think it is my mind," he answered. "The parapsychologists are always talking about the mind, but I think this power comes from somewhere outside of me, and I am just a channel for it." What did he mean by "outside"? "I believe there are other dimensions and other universes and that this energy which comes through me is coming from another universe — that it is intelligently directed and sent through me for a purpose." Puharich made assenting noises and said that what he and Uri were learning about the nature of this intelligence was astonishing.

Uri added that he thought it was very significant that all this was happening now and that people in the United States were so receptive to it. "Here is where people really believe in me and where things are going to happen." Modesty is not a Geller virtue. He described himself as "bigger than Watergate" and predicted that within a short time everyone in America would have heard of him. Already, he said, a number of high-placed American officials believed in him. The Defense Department had been especially interested in his ability to erase magnetic tapes at a distance. He described how he had made an airport TV monitor go blank in the presence of a U.S. senator. And so forth.

Uri picked up a key from the table and played with it. Everyone moved forward expectantly. "I don't know if anything will go tonight," he said. "I'm really tired and not feeling up to it." He rubbed the key with finger and thumb. "No." He dropped it. "Look, let's try some telepathy." He pointed to me. "Why don't you draw any figure on a piece of paper. I won't look." He turned his head away. I drew an infinity sign. "Now right below that draw another figure." I added a triangular pyramid. "O.K., now try to send it to me; just visualize it in your mind." Uri took up a pencil and pad. He assumed a look of concentration, first staring at me, then closing his eyes. He quickly sketched on the pad.

"The first thing I got was a circle that changed to an '8.' " He had drawn an upright "8." Underneath it he had drawn a triangle. I showed him the horizontal "8" and the pyramid. "Dammit," he said, "I saw a pyramid for an instant but then it became a triangle." I was quite impressed. "Can you send something to me?" I asked. "Oh, yes, go ahead, close your eyes." He and I both concentrated, and I came up with an ice-cream cone, possibly because I had been thinking about ice cream a lot that day. Uri had been trying to send me a sketch of a boat.

He tried a few more drawings with other people in the room and generally scored well. Then he began to miss. "There's something not right about the energy in this room," he complained.

"Can you try the key?" someone asked.

"I'll try," he replied, "but I don't think I can do it." He picked up a thick key and began stroking the shaft. Nothing happened. He placed it in his palm and tapped it with a finger. Nothing happened. "Maybe if it were lying on something metal," he suggested. A frying pan was brought. He turned it upside down and placed the key on it. He jiggled the key and tapped it, but still there was no change. "No, it's not working. Let's wait." Uri seemed a little edgy now. Every once in a while he conversed in Hebrew with Jascha Katz. Some of the guests drifted back into the other room for drinks.

"Do you only have power over metal objects?" I asked.

"Only with metals," he answered.

"Does it make any difference what kind of metal?"

"No, all metals are the same."

"Do you do any kinds of meditation or have periods of being in trance?"

"No, I'm very ordinary."

"Do you use any drugs?"

"No, not even alchhol."

"How do people react when they see you do something that's not supposed to happen?"

"Oh, man, it blows their minds. Most people are really excited and really are turned on. Some people just don't believe it even when they see it with their own eyes. Some guy on the West Coast wrote that I had a laser beam concealed in my belt. Can you imagine that?" He laughed and shook his head. "A few people believe in what I do and think it's evil."

"What do you mean?" I asked.

"Well, like that business with the projector on the plane yesterday. The stewardess was really flustered because she said that never happens. I told her it often happens when I'm on planes. I didn't mean it; it just happened. So then some of the passengers recognized me from television, and I bent a few forks for them. And then this big guy from Hawaii came over and identified himself as the security officer. It was very far out. He didn't know what to make of it. So finally he relaxed, but then he asked me how did I know that what I was doing wasn't from the Devil. He said the old Hawaiians believed powers like that were from the Devil."

"How does that make you feel?"

"Well, it makes me feel strange. I have these powers and they just come through me. I want to show them to people. I want people to know that it's real, that there are no lasers in my belt and no chemicals that I am putting on anything. I just say to the key, 'Bend!' and I just feel that it's going to bend, and it does."

"I imagine that could be heavy for some people."

"Sure, it's heavy for them. But, look, I am not a Moses or a Jesus or a messiah or anything. I believe in God, and I think that everything comes from God, but I don't think this has anything to do with God."

"Do you have any effects on living things?"

"Yes. One time in a press interview in San Francisco, they gave me a rosebud, and I put it in my hand, and the bud opened."

"How about on humans: Did you ever try to heal anyone?"

"Just one time. When I was at Stanford there was this girl who had polio, and I put my hand on her leg, and it started to move for the first time in years."

"Really?"

"Yes. But that scared me. I wouldn't like to do that again."

At this point, the lawyer asked Uri if he would please try to bend a valuable old pin that belonged to his wife and was of great emotional importance for both of them. Uri said he would try later.

"I'll try the key again," Uri said to himself. He picked up the key — it was a good solid house key — and held the head of it between the thumb and forefinger of his left hand. With his right index finger he stroked the shaft of the key. I was about six inches from him, and there was good illumination. For a long time nothing seemed to happen. Then Uri suddenly shouted: "Oh, look! There it goes!" Several of us pressed closer. At first I could see nothing different about the key. But Uri insisted: "It's bending! Yes, it's bending!" Then I could see that the tip of the key was definitely curved slightly. It had been perfectly straight before.

Uri continued to rub the key. Now the bend was easily visible, and the key could be rocked back and forth when placed on a level surface. Uri put it down on the frying pan. "It will continue to bend slowly by itself," he told us. In fact, although no motion of the key was perceptible, after several minutes the bend did seem more pronounced. "Usually, they keep bending by themselves for twenty-four hours, so by tomorrow morning it will be even more bent. It's as if they have a kind of life for a short time."

Uri now felt "hot." He correctly received two drawings sealed inside opaque envelopes — one of a cross, the other of a Star of David.

The lighting director offered Uri a very heavy gold ring set with stones. Uri examined it carefully and said he would try. He asked the owner to support the ring on edge with his forefinger. Uri then held his hand over the man's hand and finger, without touching the ring. After trying out several positions of his hand, he settled into one that he seemed to like. Again, I was only a few inches from the demonstration. Suddenly the ring sagged into an oval shape. Uri exclaimed, "There! Look at that! Did you feel anything?" The owner of the ring was equally excited. "I felt a strong tingling over the whole back of my hand, definitely some sort of energy." Uri held up the ring for all to see. It was certainly not circular any longer; in fact, it would not fit back on the owner's finger. It was not warm to the touch or in any other way odd.

There was another interlude of conversation and snacking. Uri and I and the lighting director sat together in the living room. Someone came up and asked Uri to try to bend a fork. He said he did not like to work with silverware because it was too easily bendable by hand and therefore did not make as convincing a demonstration. As he spoke, he picked up the fork by the middle in a casual manner, just to play with

it. Suddenly the fork seemed to become like melting wax
and drooped over Uri's hand. "My God! Look at that!" Uri
said. "I wasn't even trying to do it." The fork was bent at a
grotesque angle. I picked it up. It was not warm and gave no
clue as to how it had reached its new shape.

I wanted to see Uri work on something of mine that I knew
was not gimmicked. The only thing I had on me of metal
was a heavy brass belt buckle. I offered it to him. "I never
work with belt buckles," Uri said flatly.

There was little doubt in my mind that I had seen genuine
psychokinesis. I left the apartment with a sense of elation. I
still wanted to see a key of my own bent.

*

For six weeks following that evening I was out of the country. When I returned in August, Uri Geller was even more
famous, and word was out that he would appear on national
television again. On the "Tonight Show" he was unable to
cause anything unusual to happen. He tried to detect telepathically one of ten metal film canisters containing water
and tried to bend nails but could not. Johnny Carson became
impatient and urged him to try other things. Uri balked, saying he could not be rushed. It was painful to watch. At the
last minute he claimed that he produced a slight bend in a
spoon held by actor Ricardo Montalban. The camera did not
show it well, and Carson said he could not see it. A few
nights later, on the "Merv Griffin Show," Uri bent a large
nail very successfully. Griffin introduced him by saying that
the failure on the "Tonight Show" proved that Uri was real.
After all, a stage magician would succeed every time. One of
the most interesting of Uri's talents is to create belief when
he fails.

In yoga philosophy, powers like telepathy and psychokinesis are called *siddhis* and are accepted as routine acquisi-
tions in the course of self-development. Patanjali, the ancient writer who first codified the principles of yoga, wrote
in his aphorisms that the siddhis may be obtained as a result
of birth (that is, of actions performed in past lives), by
means of drugs, by the power of words (that is, by the pro-

longed repetition of certain sacred syllables or phrases), by the practice of austerities, or by the development of concentration.

If Uri Geller is a man of siddhis, he must have acquired them as a result of meritorious work in previous lives. He certainly does not practice austerities, has never used drugs, does not engage in any spiritual disciplines, and says he has no interest in meditation because he cannot sit still for more than a few seconds.

After I saw Uri perform his miracles on the Upper West Side, when I was fairly sure his powers were genuine, I began to worry about him. According to masters of yoga and other systems that acknowledge the reality of siddhis, these extraordinary mental powers are very dangerous to their possessors. In particular, they tempt one into using them for self-centered purposes — such as the acquisition of wealth or control of other persons — goals considered unhealthy from the spiritual point of view. True magic, the conscious manipulation of reality by psychic means, becomes black magic when practiced by someone who has not purified himself of ego.

Uri Geller makes no secret of his personal ambition. He speaks of his success in Israel as "small-time" and says he has come to this country to make a great deal of money and convince everyone of his powers. Listening to him talk that way, I fear for him.

One danger is that he might make some bad enemies. He told me himself that some people believe in his powers but consider them evil. Other people simply do not want to see metal objects bend in response to mental commands. A young doctor I know told me, "I don't want to know about that. It challenges all of my understanding of how the universe works." But Uri is going to show people what he can do, all the people he can, whether they want to see it or not.

He himself says he has poor control over what he does. Things happen sometimes when he does not intend them to and sometimes do not happen when he wants them to. By putting himself in positions where he has to produce phenomena on demand, he must be tempted to resort to trickery to satisfy his paying audiences.

The possibility that Uri Geller might be nothing but a trickster did not enter my mind for some time. When it did, it came by way of an amazing man named James (The Amazing) Randi, a stage magician and escape artist, who lives in New Jersey and is well known in New York from a radio show he used to do. I heard that The Amazing Randi was out to expose Uri Geller as nothing but a stage magician and that he could duplicate most of Geller's demonstrations. I thought that was worth a phone call at least.

When I told Randi I was writing an article about Uri, he was only too happy to tell me his views. "That guy is dangerous," he said. "He's a good magician, nothing more, and he's going to go on a messiah trip or get into psychic healing. That's what bothers me."

I told Randi what I had seen Uri do.

"Of course, it looks real. That's the point of magic," he said.

"But how could Uri have bent the keys?" I asked.

"He didn't," Randi replied, "they were bent already. He just reveals the bend by sleight-of-hand movements that make you think it's bending."

That did not sound very convincing. After all, I had seen the key when it was straight, and I had seen it in the process of bending. "What about the scientific tests?" I asked.

"Scientists are the people least qualified to detect chicanery," he told me. "They're the easiest to fool of all. If you want to catch a burglar, you go to a burglar, not to a scientist. If you want to catch a magician, go to a magician."

That sounded reasonable.

"Do you want to know why Geller couldn't do anything on the 'Tonight Show?' " Randi went on. "Because Carson used to be a stage magician, and I got to Carson, and we figured out exactly how to safeguard the props that were going to be used. All Geller needs is thirty seconds alone with those props and he can tamper with them. But we fixed him good."

"Well," I said, "I want to see Geller do some more of his stuff, preferably alone and with objects of my own."

"Go ahead," Randi said. "Just remember: He's good, and he knows how to fool people."

"O.K.," I said. "And maybe after I've seen some more, I'd like to visit you and see what you can do."

"Anytime," Randi agreed. "I'd really like to see the truth on this come out in the open."

My conversation with The Amazing Randi left me a little confused. I could not really see how Uri had produced the effects I saw by means of trickery unless he had accomplices in the room who supplied him with phony keys and rings. Uri certainly did not have the manner of a magician. Also, I know that stage magicians are the worst skeptics around. Because they do everything by trickery, they see trickery everywhere. Randi, for example, thought psychic healing was always fraud. But what if Uri Geller were a fake? What would that say about the Stanford Research Institute and other scientific experts who had backed him and were thinking up explanations of the mysterious "energy" he uses? What would that say about my own credulity?

A few days later I met with Uri privately in his apartment. I told him I wanted to see more of him and hoped he would not mind if I tagged along at some of his performances. He said he would not. I asked him what he thought about people who said he was a magician.

"I am not a magician," he said vehemently. "Look, the people who are supposed to see these things will see them, and those who don't, don't. I don't care if people say I do magic tricks. I know that it's real. And it's all good publicity." He was charming, as usual, and very unmagicianlike.

Later I traveled to Houston and Austin, but because of a mix-up in travel arrangements, I arrived in both cities a few hours after Uri had left. The only evidence I found of his visit was a front-page story in *The Daily Texan*, The University of Texas newspaper. It read in part:

> During an interview Wednesday, Geller, in town for his second performance here in three months, bent a heavy metal key to al-

most a forty-five degree angle by stroking it lightly. When he slid a steel spoon through a circle formed by his fingers, the spoon began to bend visibly. He then set the utensil on the carpet at his feet, where it continued to bend the better part of an hour without anyone or anything touching it further.

The *Texan* reporter and photographer present could see no possible way the Israeli psychic could have used fakery to bend the objects.*

*

At the end of September, Uri Geller appeared before a capacity audience at Town Hall in New York City. By now, articles about him had appeared in still more periodicals, including *The New Scientist* in London. Almost all of these stories took him at face value — as a gifted psychic come to demonstrate the reality of mind over matter. I heard his name invoked to bolster the claims of various groups that a new age was upon us. Nevertheless, *New York Magazine* suggested Uri was a fraud and quoted The Amazing Randi in support of that position. Meanwhile, more and more Geller stories were in circulation. Edgar Mitchell — former astronaut, ESP buff, and Geller backer — made it known that Uri was going to try to teleport a camera back to earth from the moon, where Mitchell had left it. Dr. Puharich described some of the more spectacular materializations he had seen Uri perform and hinted that Uri had been in communication with intelligent beings in flying saucers. Stanford Research Institute was going to do more controlled studies of Uri. Bell Laboratories might work with him, too.

In the midst of this swirl of stories, the Town Hall appearance was disappointing. Puharich gave his usual introduction, then Uri appeared and asked for everyone to be with him. He launched the show with the same demonstrations of telepathy I had seen him do last spring in Berkeley, guessing a color written on a blackboard (blue) and a capital city (Denver). Then he tried something different. He had one woman volunteer write a color on the blackboard (it was purple), and he attempted to receive this color telepathically

* September 20, 1973.

from the audience and project it to a second woman volunteer standing next to him. After several tries he shook his head. "No, I'm not getting anything."

"Ask her if she got anything," someone called out.

"No, it's not working," Uri said. "I'm just getting confused impressions."

"Ask her anyway," several people shouted.

"O.K., what did you receive?" Uri asked the woman standing next to him.

"I got purple," she answered. There was a loud cheer from the audience.

"Sometimes it happens that way," Uri said. "When people are around me, their telepathic powers come out. It's like when I'm on television, the stations are getting hundreds of calls from people who say that spoons and forks are bending in their homes while I'm on. Just last week I heard that in the Texas attorney general's office in Austin, a secretary was listening to a tape of a radio show I did there and a fork started to bend in the presence of four witnesses."

After completing the telepathy portion of the show, Uri asked for questions and talked a lot about himself. He waxed defiant at several points and, particularly, lashed out at critics who said he should not be turning his powers to use in stage performances.

"Look, it's my life," he said, "and nobody is going to tell me how to live it. If I want to make money, I am going to make money." This brought a round of applause. But the talk went on and on, and the audience grew restless. By the time Uri was ready to start repairing stopped watches, people were not with him as much as they had been. Perhaps for that reason, he could not get a single watch to run, though he tried working on many.

He attempted to bend rings but could not do that either. People in the audience shouted out suggestions. Uri ran through a great many rings and a great many women volunteers without success. Finally, at the very end, he tried concentrating on two rings at once and caused one with a zodiac insignia to pop apart. A televised image of the ring was projected onto a screen above the stage for all to see. With that, Uri ended the show. The audience appeared pleased.

Three days later I went again to Uri's apartment, this time equipped with several keys; a long, threaded steel bolt; and a stopped watch. The watch had not run for a long time. If jarred, it would go for about five seconds and stop. When I got to the apartment, five others were present: four people from *Rolling Stone* and a reporter from Boston's *Real Paper*. I walked into the middle of an intense session. The table was littered with bent spoons, a bent key, a gold ring on a piece of paper, a watch, many papers with drawings of geometrical figures, and tape recorders. Everyone was very animated.

Uri seemed tired but enthusiastic. He told me to ask him anything. I said I'd prefer to sit and listen for a time. The talk focused on flying saucers and astral projection but also included many questions I'd heard Uri asked before. One of the *Rolling Stone* men asked if Uri could teach others to do the things he does. "How can I?" he answered. "Where would I begin?" I asked him if there were any verification of the bendings reported by home viewers of his television appearances. "Oh, yes," he replied and repeated the story of the fork in the attorney general's office in Austin, Texas. "And that was just with a tape of a radio show!" I suggested that these occurrences, if true, might represent the mobilization of the psychokinetic abilities of other persons. Uri agreed. He also talked about reports of broken watches starting to run again in the homes of people watching him on television.

A woman from *Rolling Stone* told me that he had fixed the watch on the table just by holding his hand over it. The *Real Paper* man reached for the watch to show it to me and suddenly became excited. "Has anyone reset this?" he asked. Everyone looked at the watch and gasped. Apparently it was now four hours ahead of where it had been. Uri picked it up and exclaimed, "My God! Look at that!" He put it down. Moments later it had advanced again. "It's always like that," Uri explained. "You never see the hands moving. You just find them in a new position."

I said I had a broken watch with me, but even as I drew it out of my pocket, I had a funny feeling that it would be going. And so it was — quite steadily. Uri took credit for this, even though he had not known the watch had been in my pocket. Had he mobilized my latent psychokinetic ability? I wondered to myself. We set both watches to the correct time and left them side by side to see what would happen.

The *Rolling Stone* people told me the ring on the piece of paper had levitated earlier, or at least, it had dropped out of midair onto the table. No one had seen how it got to a position in midair. They had seen a key bend, and there had been much guessing correctly of drawings made out of Uri's sight. I took out of my pocket my collection of keys and my long bolt and put them amid the clutter on the table, hoping Uri would consent to work on them. The bolt rolled a little, I think because I bumped the table. "Who moved that?" Uri asked, very excited, grabbing me by the shoulder. "Did you touch that?" I said I did not know, and it became another miracle. Miracles were happening right and left.

"Let's try an experiment by phone," Uri suggested to me. "Call up someone you know, and I'll try to send him a number." I called up a friend, the owner of the broken watch I had borrowed for the afternoon. I told him his watch was fixed and asked him to try to think of the number between one and ten that Uri Geller was trying to send him. Just then, Jascha Katz, one of Uri's promoters, came into the room to say that Uri had a call from Paris on another phone. Uri left. The phone I was holding went dead. When Uri came back, I told him the phone was dead. "My God!" he exclaimed, "I hope I didn't knock him out." But another call discovered my friend alive and well and dimly thinking of the number three. Uri had been sending "7" (he had written it down) but showed us that he had first written "3" and crossed it out.

I asked if he would try to bend one of my keys. He took up a short brass one. "O.K., I'll try, but don't be disappointed if it doesn't work. I'm very tired and I don't know whether I can do it now." He stroked the key while I hunched over him. Nothing happened, "No, I'm too tired. Maybe later."

The mood became manic, and the *Rolling Stone* people began to get headaches. "There's a lot of energy in this room," one of them said.

Uri asked me to shoot a roll of film of him using one of the reporters' cameras with the lens cap on. "I'll try to make images come out on the film." He held his hands in strange positions in front of the covered lens and assumed looks of great concentration as I went through the roll. "I think I may have done it," he announced.

Then more people came in: the director of the Channel 5 news show and Martin Abend, the political commentator for Channel 5. The director had spent the early part of the afternoon with Uri and was now a solid convert. Uri had detected metal in film cans, caused a key to bend, and done much successful ESP. Channel 5 was going to do a feature on Uri that night and wanted Martin Abend to comment afterward. Abend seemed unsure of all this. "It's not my line," he kept saying. But the director assured him that he would have an amazing experience if he would just suspend his doubts and watch. "But if it is real, I can't say that over the air," Abend protested. "Do you know what kind of a storm we'd stir up?" He frowned. The *Rolling Stone* people urged him to be open-minded and told him proudly that they had always been believers. "Just try to help him, you'll see." Then the five reporters left, leaving me with Uri, Martin Abend, and the news director. The director was very keyed up, anxious for Uri to convince Abend as he had been convinced earlier. They tried some simple ESP. Abend drew a geometrical figure and Uri looked away, then tried to reproduce the figure while Abend concentrated on it. Uri did not do very well. Then he tried to bend a key and did not succeed. Finally, he sent the news director away: "You're making me nervous."

Abend and Geller tried more drawings with equivocal results. Uri tried sending drawings to Abend. "Come on," Abend said, "I don't have any ESP power." They tried, and again the results were equivocal. Then Abend drew two intersecting circles. Uri received, first, two circles tangent to each other, then two circles, one inside the other. Abend was impressed. "That's really something," he said. "I can do much better when I'm not tired," Uri told him. "No, that's *good*," Abend replied. There was another unsuccessful attempt at key bending. The television people took their leave, telling us the show would be on at ten o'clock on the evening news, only a few hours away.

Uri and I were now alone, sitting together on a couch. I told him I hated to ask him to perform again, but I had really never seen him bend anything of mine and had to do so before I could report that he did it. "Let's try the key again," he suggested. We did, but with no luck. "What else do you have?" he asked. I brought out two other keys on a small chain attached to a little knife. "I used to have a knife like that," he said and put it into my hand. He covered it with my other hand, then put his hands on mine. He concentrated intently but to no effect. Then he looked at the other keys and asked which I was most attached to. I was not sure. He piled all the keys into my hand and added the knife on top. Then he repeated the operation. I felt a pulsation and told him so, but there was no change.

"Dammit!" he said. "Why can't I do anything?"

"Don't be disappointed," I told him. "I'm very patient, and if nothing works now, there will be another time."

Uri seemed wrought up. "Don't you have anything else metal?" he asked. "Maybe in your boots." He pointed to my boots that I had left across the room. I looked at them.

"No, all I've got is a belt buckle, and you told me once you never worked with belt buckles."

"Let's try it," he said. I took off my belt and put the large brass buckle in my palm on top of the three keys and the knife and chain. I covered the pile with my other hand. Uri put his hand on top. More intense concentration. Suddenly, I felt a distinct throb inside my hands, like a small frog kicking. I told him so. "You did?" he asked excitedly and opened my hands. I could see no change in the buckle. He pulled out a long steel key and cried out, "It's bent, yes, it's bent! Do you see?" I did not see at first. But then I did notice a slight bend. It was very exciting. Uri put the key on the table to check it. Yes, it was definitely bent.

Uri was almost jumping up and down for joy, and I shared his emotion. "Let's see if we can bend it more," he said. He touched the key to the other keys, stroked it again. After a few minutes the bend was about twenty-five degrees. Uri patted me on the back, making me feel that I had participated in the miracle. "It's good you felt it jump, man," he told me. "Not many people can feel that." I was elated.

He ran into the other room to tell Jascha Katz of the success, then hugged me warmly. I gathered up my things, thanking him profusely and telling him I had seen exactly what I wanted. He walked me to the elevator. As we were saying good-bye, there was a *plink!* and the long steel bolt I had brought bounced off his left arm onto the floor. "Is this something of yours?" he asked, picking it up. "Yes," I said, "I brought it along but must have left it inside." His eyes widened. "My God! Just like their ring. You've just seen a materialization!" He grew even more excited and rushed back inside to tell Jascha the latest. Somehow, I was less moved by the materializing bolt than by the bending key. It could so easily have been a sleight-of-hand trick.

In any case, I left his apartment a convert and hurried back to dinner with friends. "I have no doubt that Uri Geller is real," I announced. Then we watched the Channel 5 news. There was Uri again, in a very long segment, bending a key, getting drawings, locating metal hidden in cans. The reporters presented him as unquestionably real: There was "no possibility" that he could have deceived them. Then came a round-table discussion with the reporters, Martin Abend, and a professional magician out to discredit Uri. The magician came off badly. He did not believe in psychic phenomena and said Geller had to be a phony. Abend defended Geller by recounting his own experience with him.

"I drew two intersecting circles," Abend told the magician, "and tried to send them to Geller. Now I think that's an unusual sort of figure. Geller first drew two circles tangent to one another. Then he drew two intersecting circles. It was an amazing thing."

I noted with interest that Abend had not reported this incident correctly. In fact, Uri had come closer with the tangent circles. His second attempt had been one circle inside another. Initially a skeptic, Abend had remembered what happened in a way that made Uri look better.

I called several friends to tell them of my evening with Uri and my new faith in him. In a way I was sorry I had made an appointment to see The Amazing Randi at his house in New Jersey the following day. After all, what could he possibly show me that would change my mind?

*

The Amazing Randi lives in a house guarded by two beautiful macaws. On the door is a Peruvian mask from which blaring martial music issues when the bell is rung. The door opens from the opposite side one would expect from the position of the doorknob. Inside are mummy cases, clocks that run backwards, and other strange objects that plainly advertise the dweller as a creator of illusions.

I met Randi less than twenty-four hours after I had become a Geller convert and when I was still feeling good about my experience of the previous evening.

Randi turned out to be a delightful host, talkative and funny, with a twinkle in his eye and a roguish look to let you know that he might be up to fooling you. I told Randi what I had seen Uri do. He listened attentively but made no comments. When I finished, he invited me over to a table on which were envelopes, paper, nails, nuts, bolts, and little aluminum film canisters, the sort that rolls of 35-millimeter film come in.

"What shall we try first?" he asked. "Some telepathy?" He invited me to take a piece of paper and three envelopes. "Go to the other end of the room or out of the room," he instructed. "Draw any figure you like on the paper, fold it up, seal it in an envelope, seal that envelope in another envelope, and that in the third." I followed the instructions and brought the sealed envelope back. Deep inside was a drawing of two intersecting circles.

"We'll put that aside for now," Randi said, setting it down

on the table. He handed me a carton of sturdy four-inch nails. "Pick any six that you think are perfectly straight." I did. I also looked to make sure they were real nails. "Now put a rubber band around that bunch and set them aside." I did.

"Meanwhile, let's try one of Mr. Geller's favorite tricks." Randi picked ten film canisters and told me to stuff one of them full of nuts and bolts — "so tightly that it won't rattle if moved." He went out of the room while I did this. "Now mix them all up," he shouted from the kitchen. When I had done so, Randi came back and sat down at the table.

He studied the canisters and moved his hand over them without touching them. "I'm going to eliminate the empty ones," he told me. "When I point to one and say it's empty, you remove it. And set it down quietly so I can't tell anything from the sound." He made passes over the canisters, just as I had seen Uri Geller do on television. "That one's empty," he said confidently pointing to a canister in the middle. I removed it and set it aside. "Don't tell me if I'm wrong," he said. "That one's empty." He pointed to another. Randi had a great sense of drama, and I found myself very involved with his performance. He eliminated another canister and another. Finally, only two were left. He passed his palm over one and then the other as if feeling for subtle emanations from the metal inside. "That's empty," he said at last, indicating the one on the left. I removed it. It was empty. The remaining can was full of nuts and bolts. He had never touched the canisters nor jarred the table. I was amazed.

"Now," Randi told me, "that was a trick. And I'm going to show you how to do it. But I want you to promise you won't reveal the method, because magicians aren't supposed to reveal secrets. This is a special case." I gave my promise, and Randi taught me how he did it. It was very simple — so simple a child could master it. In fact, Randi said he had taught several children to do it. The trick is based on a subtle but easily perceptible difference between the full can and the empty ones — a difference that can be seen at once if you know what to look for.

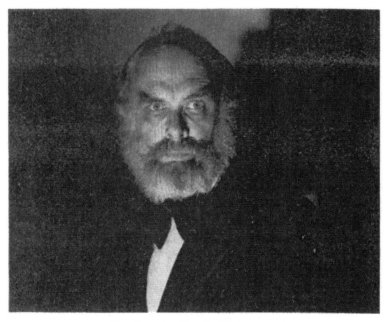

The Amazing Randi. (Kriegsmann)

"What if the canister is filled with water?" I asked.

"It's the same idea; you just look for different things. Do you remember when Mr. Geller tried to do that on the 'Tonight Show'?" Randi asked. I thought I did. "Let's look at it," he said. Randi has a videotape machine in his house and recordings of most of Uri Geller's television appearances. "I learned how he does most of his tricks by studying these tapes," he explained. We relived the famous "Tonight Show." There was Johnny Carson telling Uri to go ahead and do something. There were the film canisters, one full of water. Uri stalled. "We handled those cans in a way that eliminated the difference," Randi said. Uri was moving his hand over the canisters. "No, I'm not getting it," he said and gave up.

We sat through the rest of the show in which nothing happened. "Now look at this," Randi said. He put on a videotape of the "Merv Griffin Show," where Uri had appeared a few nights later. The high point of that show was the bending of a nail.

"All right, back to the table," Randi said. He picked up the bunch of six nails. "Let's find one that's absolutely straight." He rolled each one back and forth on the table, keeping up a constant patter while eliminating those nails that had what he called "little woggily-woggilies" — slight irregularities that kept them from rolling smoothly. He ended up with one nail that he liked, holding it between thumb and forefinger, midway along the shaft. "Now, keep your eye on it," he said, "I'm going to try to bend it." He rolled it back and forth slowly and gently between his thumb and forefinger. I hardly knew what to expect. Suddenly, the nail began to bend before my eyes. "Look at that," Randi chuckled. Sure enough: It was bent to about thirty degrees.

I shook my head in astonishment. "Not bad, huh?" Randi asked. I allowed as how it was not bad. I took the nail. It was not warm or in any way unusual. Just bent. Then, also before my eyes, Randi showed me in slow motion how he had substituted a bent nail for one of the straight ones, how he had concealed the bend from me until the proper moment, then revealed it while rubbing the nail between his fingers. I had seen it bend. Suddenly, I experienced a sense of how strongly the mind can impose its own interpretation on perceptions: how it can see what it expects to see and not see what it does not expect to see.

"Now, let's watch that tape of the 'Merv Griffin Show' again and see how Uri does it," Randi suggested. Sure enough, there was Uri Geller manipulating three nails just as Randi had. Under Randi's tutelage, I could see that one nail was never, in fact, shown in its entirety to the close-up camera, even though Uri was claiming to hold up each nail, one at a time, to prove its straightness.

"Ready for some more telepathy?" Randi asked. "Let's try that sealed envelope." He went back to the table, sat down, pulled up a pad and pen, and held the envelope to his forehead. "You concentrate on the figure," he told me. He started making marks on the paper and drew out an equals sign. He seemed to be way off. "Now don't tell me how I'm doing," he said, "just let me work on it." Slowly, he ex-

tended the lines, crossing them into a flat X. All the time he
muttered to himself. Then the lines began to curve. "Oh, I
see it now," he said happily. And there on the pad appeared
the two intersecting circles, exactly as I had drawn them.
There was no doubt that Randi had known what was in the
envelope. I opened the envelopes, one by one, took out the
folded paper, and showed it to him. "Well, well," he said,
pleased with himself. "Look at that."

Randi showed me how he did that one, too, and it was also
very simple. Really, there is only one way to know what is
inside an envelope without using powers, and that way involves getting your hands on the envelope for a while. "People come back from seeing Uri Geller," Randi said, "and
they say, 'He never touched the envelope,' but if you question them carefully, what they really mean is: He never
touched it in ways that they think would have enabled him
to know what was inside. That is the basis of stage magic.
You take advantage of little opportunities to do the dirty
work and know that people aren't going to notice you. Geller
is a master opportunist."

"Have you ever seen him doing the dirty work?" I asked.

"I sure have. I was at Town Hall the other night. The thing
that irks me is how much people let him get away with —
things they wouldn't let a magician get away with. Remember when he asked that woman to write a foreign capital on the blackboard, and she wrote 'Denver?' The whole
audience was annoyed at her for not following instructions.
At one point, every head turned to glare at her, and right
then old Uri just shot a glance at the blackboard. It's that
simple. When he broke that ring at the end — remember
that? He said, 'Let's try two rings at once.' What he did was
click off his microphone for an instant, wedge one ring into
the other, and give a hard squeeze so that the zodiac ring
broke where the setting was joined."

"You saw that?"

"I saw it. It's that simple. Everybody looks for complicated explanations, and the explanations are always simple.
That's why you don't see them. The people who are easiest
to take in with that sort of thing are intelligent people, espe-

cially scientists. The people who are hard to fool are the feeble-minded, because they look at what they're not supposed to look at. Scientists are pushovers."

"Has the Stanford Research Institute ever had a professional magician act as a consultant in their studies of Geller?" I asked.

"Never! Isn't that unbelievable? They get insulted if you suggest it, or they say that a magician would put out 'bad vibes' that would interfere with Uri's abilities."

"All right," I said. "I'm convinced by everything you've showed me and told me. But last night Uri Geller bent one of my keys for me. Can you do the same?"

"Got a key?" Randi asked. I brought out the brass key that Uri had failed to bend. "Give it to me." Randi took the key and played with it for a while. "Yes, I think that will work," he said. He sat down across from me and held the key under my nose, rubbing it between his thumb and forefinger.

"Look at that," he said. "I think it's going." The key was bending. In a trice it was bent to about thirty degrees, looking for all the world like a Geller production.

"No!" I protested. My faith in Uri Geller lay in pieces on the floor.

"All I needed was a moment in which your attention was distracted to bend the key by jamming it against my chair. I made the bend appear just as I did with the nail." Again I had seen not just a bend but actual bending.

"Have you ever tried to bend a key with your hands?" Randi asked.

"A little. I've just assumed I couldn't."

Randi then showed me how he could bend a key with his hands. I was able to do the same, although with difficulty. I saw that with practice one could get very good at bending metal objects quickly and surreptitiously without recourse to lasers concealed in the belt or other complicated devices.

Randi also made a fork bend for me, although he could not simulate the fork I had seen melt over Uri's hand.* He astounded me with other sleight-of-hand tricks. Even when I

---

* Randi has since claimed that he can now reproduce this effect as well.

knew what to look for, I could not see him doing the "dirty work."

"Do you think that knowing what I do now, I could see Geller doing it?"

"I doubt it," Randi replied. "He's very good. He can take advantage of any situation and turn it to his credit. People want to believe in him."

I remembered how Martin Abend had improved upon Uri's telepathic performance and how I had embellished some of what I had seen in telling others about it.

"What about the time I saw him make a ring sag into an oval shape without touching it?" I asked.

"Look, I can't explain all of what he does, especially if I haven't seen it. I repeat: He's good. And he probably has many different techniques available. But if an accomplished professional has a chance to watch him closely, it can all be figured out. That's why Uri won't go anywhere near me or any other magician."

"How did you get a chance to watch him up close?"

"First by masquerading as a reporter when he was interviewed at *Time* and then by studying the videotapes."

"Do you want to expose him?"

"I'd love to, but I don't think that will be easy. The fact that I can duplicate his feats by magic tricks proves nothing. The only way would be to catch him substituting a bent nail or jamming a key against a chair leg, and that will be difficult."

I thanked The Amazing Randi for his time and went on my way, amazed. I had never before had the experience of going from such total belief to such total disbelief in so short a time. Nor had I ever doubted my perceptions so thoroughly.

Since then I have thought a lot about Uri Geller and have talked with others about him. One person I spoke to was Ray Hyman, a professor of psychology at the University of Oregon in Eugene, who teaches a course called "The Pseudopsychologies." It deals with astrology and various psychic and occult phenomena. Dr. Hyman describes himself as an "open-minded skeptic, who has never seen a genuine psychic phenomenon" and does not know what kind of evidence it would take to convince him of the existence of such things. He has a background in stage magic and spent a day at the Stanford Research Institute watching Uri Geller in December 1972. He decided that Uri was "a very good magician and an incredible opportunist" and that he could replicate most of what he saw by simple tricks.

"What I find most interesting about Uri Geller are the reactions to him," Hyman told me. "For instance, the physicists at Stanford were irate at the suggestion that Geller might be tricking them. They were physicists — real scientists — and I was only a psychologist. I was astounded that they had never bothered to check up on Uri's background in Israel."

Hyman showed me correspondence from a professor of psychology at the Hebrew University of Jerusalem who described Uri's early work as a stage magician and enclosed clippings from Israeli papers denouncing Geller as a fraud. At one point, an Israeli court ordered him to refund money to a man who contended that he had produced magic tricks and not psychic phenomena, as advertised for his performance.

"The questions of whether he's real or not is less interesting than what he's showing us about the nature of evidence and the way belief shapes perception," Hyman went on. "Uri Geller is an important person. We can learn a lot from him." I agree.

*

Publication of the original newsletters on Uri Geller as a two-part article in *Psychology Today* put me in the enemy camp as far as Uri Geller's friends were concerned. At the same time, a psychologist attacked me in print for having been taken in by Geller. You can't win.

I have seen Uri Geller only once since 1973. In September 1975 he was the star attraction at a strange event called the First World Congress of Sorcery, held in Bogotá, Colombia. I was there also, having been invited to give a lecture on "The Positive Use of Magic Plants." The congress was a sort of cross between a commercial exposition and a psychic ex-

travaganza, complete with witch doctors, researchers, sensation seekers, and assorted eccentrics. Uri was a great hit,
bending forks and fixing watches, both in person and on
Colombian national television. The Colombians were completely at his feet. No one suggested that trickery might be
involved.

Since then, Uri's star has waned. The days of major television appearances and standing-room-only crowds seem to be
gone. Many of the scientists who vouched for his abilities
have withdrawn their support, and the Stanford Research
Institute is a bit embarrassed about the whole affair. The
public has certainly lost interest.

What is there to conclude from this maddeningly contradictory mass of data?

I think the question of whether Uri Geller is real or not is
essentially unanswerable. As deep as I got into trying to answer that question, the only conclusion I came up with was:
maybe yes, maybe no. I cannot say with certainty that Uri
Geller does not have any of the powers he claims. I have an
intuitive conviction that such powers exist. I also have a
strong feeling that Uri is mainly a brilliantly artistic stage
magician, whose ability to create belief is great. I am not to-
tally sure, however, that stage magic can explain all that I
saw him do. That is as far as I can go without getting very
confused.

In my wanderings through this hall of mirrors I noted
some interesting similarities among the main characters.
For example, when I was around both Uri Geller and James
Randi, I found that my mood brightened and my thinking
was stimulated. In their own ways, both of them showed me
very clearly that my sense impressions of reality are not necessarily the same as reality, and I value that experience. Uri
believes in psychic phenomena, and The Amazing Randi
does not. They balance each other nicely: Uri's excesses of
belief (his preoccupations with intelligences outside the universe, for example) complement Randi's excesses of skep-
ticism ("Psychic healing is a bunch of nonsense").

People who believe in telepathy and psychokinesis are

sometimes accused of thinking wishfully. I have always thought that people who denied the existence of such things were also thinking wishfully — that is, ignoring certain kinds of evidence while paying attention to others. Leon Jaroff, the editor of *Time* who wrote the negative story about Uri Geller, is quoted in *New York Magazine* as saying, "There has never been a single adequately documented 'psychic phenomenon.' Many people believe in things like this because they need to." That view discounts completely the evidence of direct experience. It, too, is based on a need to see things a certain way.

Selective perception of evidence is the basic method by which we construct our models of reality. Many systems of thought urge us to distinguish between reality and our models of it. For example, one of the important themes in don Juan's philosophy as transmitted by Carlos Castaneda is that what we call "objective" reality is nothing more than a consistent model — one of many possible — built up of learned and habitual ways of selecting evidence and interpreting perceptions.

Some of these systems go on to suggest that human imagination, and particularly the capacity to fantasize, are vitally involved in the process of shaping reality and making it seem objective. "Wishful thinking," though it has a negative connotation, is an appropriate term for this process, and we all engage in it, often unconsciously, to bring things into reality according to our needs and to make them leave reality according to our needs.

That is why questions like, Do psychic phenomena exist? are unanswerable. The answer is always yes and no, depending on who is looking from what point of view. Each of us has the power to make such phenomena real in our lives or not. The first step toward making them real is to believe that evidence exists. In this way, "faith" or "wishful thinking" is a technique used to obtain certain experiences that make the technique unnecessary thereafter.

18

WHEN THE SUN DIES

ONCE, I SAW PEOPLE APPLAUD the sky. They were Mexican villagers and Indians crowded into the market town of Mia-huatlán in Oaxaca state on a cloudless Saturday morning in March 1970, and they broke into their spontaneous ovation for the heavens at twenty-seven minutes before noon. At that moment the edge of the sun peered out from behind the moon, where it had been in total eclipse for three minutes and twenty-nine seconds. The applause was not so much a welcome to the reappearing sun as a joyful thank-you to na-ture for putting on such a glorious show.

People who have seen only partial solar eclipses cannot know the beauty of the full spectacle because the experience within the path of totality is different not in degree but in kind. On that Saturday in 1970, I stood on a hill above Mia-huatlán — a hill that commanded a sweeping view of rugged, arid plains and distant mountains. For some time the light had been fading ever more quickly. Then, with great drama, a nebulous darkness grew out of the west — the edge of the umbra, or cone of shadow, whose swift passage over the globe traces the path of the total eclipse. The vast sky of southern Mexico became the dome of a giant planetarium as an unseen hand turned down a cosmic rheostat. The town of Miahuatlán became a model railroad set at my feet, and I experienced a powerful sense of what psychiatrists call "derealization" — the feeling of external things becoming unreal and weird. In the next instant, things really did get weird. Suddenly, the surface of the earth was covered by

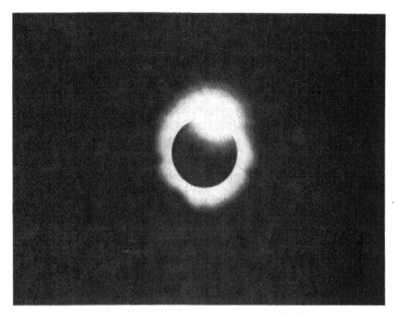

Sun's corona and diamond ring, seen during the total eclipse of March 7, 1970, at Miahuatlán, Oaxaca, Mexico. (Jay Pasachoff)

rippling bands of alternating light and shadow: patterns generated by the interaction of light rays from the last remaining points of the disappearing solar crescent with the earth's upper atmosphere. These "shadow bands" persisted for a timeless interval, absorbing my full attention. Then someone shouted, "Look!" and I turned my gaze upward and saw for the first time in my life the corona of the sun.

High in the sky, for the sun was near the zenith when the moon overtook it, was a black disc — surrounding it, a blaze of silver light of unearthly beauty. The sky was not very dark; a glowing twilight prevailed, with a 360-degree rim of light around the horizon, giving a strong impression of being under a dome. Mercury and Venus were in brilliant view, but the light of the corona was too bright for other stars to be visible. I had never seen Mercury before. There was a quality to those minutes within the umbra that must be like the feeling in the eye of a hurricane. After all the dramatic changes of accelerating intensity, everything stopped: There was an improbable sense of peace and equilibrium. Time did not flow. I have no way of comparing those three and a half minutes of clock time to any other three-and-a-half-minute interval I have experienced.

For the whole time, I gazed at the eclipsed sun with my naked eyes. (The light of the corona can do no damage to the eyes, and I would not have looked at it any other way.) Then, all at once, a spot of blinding yellow light appeared, the corona vanished in the glare, shadow bands raced across the landscape once more, and the dome of shadow melted away to the east. It was then that all of Miahuatlán broke into applause.

For hours afterward, everyone I saw on the streets wore a radiant smile. Even some of the scientists who had barricaded themselves into regimented observation posts in order to study the eclipse were transfigured. People were high, and it showed in their faces.

My experience in Miahuatlán affected me powerfully. For one thing, I became an overt eclipse freak, eager to put myself again in the path of the umbra. In Mexico I met people who had followed total solar eclipses around the earth all their lives; I now understood that passion. When I heard that a long eclipse would be visible in Africa in 1973, I resolved to be there. More than anything else, the splendor of the eclipse had impressed me. There was nothing at all terrifying — no plunge into scary blackness, as fictional accounts of eclipses would have us believe. The reaction of people in the shadow was to get high on the strangeness and beauty of the event.

Whenever an eclipse is visible in America, newspapers chuckle about Indians who think dragons are swallowing the sun. In fact, civilized Americans seem to be more peculiar about eclipses than the Indians I saw in Mexico. The path of totality of that same 1970 eclipse crossed the southeastern corner of the United States, entering the country at northwest Florida and leaving at Virginia Beach. The same newspapers that made fun of uncivilized natives carried horrifying warnings about the dangers of looking at the eclipse. Some medical experts urged the public to stay away entirely from the umbral zone, as if merely being near it were unhealthy.

Evidence of this phobia is provided by a remarkable document sent to me on my return from Mexico by a friend who worked for the U.S. Department of Justice. It is an official Justice Department document titled "Memorandum to All Employees (Legal and Administrative Activities); Subject: Safe Viewing of the Eclipse" and is dated March 2, 1970. The memorandum is signed "Charles M. Odell, Chief, Personnel Operations Section, Administrative Division." It reads as follows:

The purpose of this memorandum is to alert Department employees and their families of the impending eclipse of the sun, due Saturday, March 7th, at approximately 1:30 p.m. This fascinating but dangerous sight will last for three minutes — time to do irreparable damage to the eyes.

The eye damage hazard is due to the fact that the sun can be looked at without discomfort during an eclipse. Normally the dazzling visible rays prevent anyone from looking directly at the sun. Although the visible rays are blocked during an eclipse, the harmful, invisible infra-red rays continue to be emitted, and can cause damaging burns to the retina, the delicate inner layer of the eye which transmits images to the brain. The retina is not sensitive to pain, so a retinal burn is not "felt." But retinal burns cannot be cured, and produce a permanent blind spot in the victim's field of vision — in the vital small area used for reading and "fine" seeing.

"There is no safe way to view the eclipse directly," says the National Society for the Prevention of Blindness. "The public must be made aware that the so-called protective devices, such as sunglasses, smoked glass, or film negatives do not protect the eye from the invisible infra-red rays which do the damage."

A safe indirect method of viewing the eclipse, recommended by the Prevention of Blindness Society, is a simple projection device which can be made by taking two pieces of white cardboard, making a pinhole in one and *with the sun at your back*, focus the eclipse through the pinhole onto the second board. The size of the image can be changed by altering the distance between the boards. However, *the best way to view the eclipse is on television*.

In some newspaper articles, a variant of the cardboard projection device was suggested: The viewer was told to put the pinhole in one end of a cardboard carton and put the carton over his head; the projected image could then be viewed safely and clearly within a miniature, portable theater. This device was used by many people on the beaches of Virginia. Now, it seems to me that people who put cardboard boxes over their heads to avoid looking at the beauty of a total eclipse ought not to go around making fun of other people's beliefs about eclipses. I am not certain, but I suspect that one does not get high off an eclipse while hiding under a box, and I am pretty sure that the effect does not come through at all on television.

Warnings of this sort had great impact on the public. When I returned from Mexico and told people I had looked at the eclipse directly, many said, "You did? And you can still see?" I met people who had spent hours of anguish waiting for their sight to fail simply because they had glanced up at the sky while driving during the height of the partial eclipse in New York and Boston. It is true that careless staring at the crescent sun during the partial phase of a solar eclipse can lead to a retinal burn, but the most elementary precautions (such as using exposed film and looking at the sun in brief glimpses) reduce this risk to zero. I repeat that one can look with the unprotected eye for the entire period of totality. There is no medical justification for telling people not to watch eclipses.

I was curious to know why the medical profession had spread such fear and why the Justice Department had bothered itself about a solar eclipse. Are eclipses dangerous in some way to the established order of society?

I think they may be, and to get more information on that possibility I placed myself within the path of totality of the solar eclipse of June 30, 1973. The shadow of that eclipse crossed the Atlantic from the northeast corner of South America to the coast of Mauritania, swept across central Africa, and found me in a Gabra camp in the middle of the Chalbi Desert in Kenya's Northern Frontier District. The

Chalbi is a baked wasteland of intense heat, wild winds, and occasional waterholes. For at least four years it had been in the grip of a killing drought that showed no signs of letting up. The people who lived there were near the edge of starvation. The Gabra are a nomadic tribe of camel herders who move their camps every few weeks in search of forage for their livestock. They live in small round huts constructed of hides on frames of interlaced poles. When the camp is ready to move, the women take the huts apart and pack them onto the camels.

The camp I was in had twenty huts arranged in a straight line, their doors facing west. In back of this row of homes were several small corrals made of thornbush in which young camels were kept while their parents were driven each day to water or forage. There was no other sign of human presence on the desert landscape. Each day the Gabra had to walk several hours to Maikona, a well complex, to water their animals and fill their water jars. Each morning before sunrise the herdboys went off with a parade of camels, and each evening around sunset they returned.

The people of this tiny settlement worked hard all the time merely to survive in their hostile environment. There were no days of rest, no letups in the daily routine of milking the camels, leading them to food and water, and collecting water for the camp. At the time of my arrival, these Gabra had eaten no meat in many weeks and no cornmeal in a month. Even in times of plenty they do not eat fish, fowl, fruit, or vegetables. Now, in a time of great hardship, they were surviving on camel milk and tea.

I arrived in the camp two days before the eclipse, along with an anthropologist, three other Americans, and two translators — high school boys of Gabra origin who spoke English, Swahili, and Gabra, although they had grown up in towns and never lived in traditional Gabra camps. We were part of a larger expedition to study the impact of the eclipse on the Borana — a cattle-herding people of northern Kenya and southern Ethiopia who intermingle with the Gabra. The Borana have a sophisticated cosmology that attributes great significance (mostly negative) to eclipses. Most of our group was scattered in Borana camps on the fringes of the Marsabit National Reserve, an island of green adjoining the Chalbi Desert. The Borana looked sleeker than the Gabra and certainly were living on better land. I chose to be out in the Chalbi mainly because the desert landscape seemed better for eclipse viewing. I was interested more in the sun than in either the Borana or Gabra and was willing to endure the hostility of the Chalbi for a better show.

The chief of our camp, a handsome man named Duba who had once served in the native colonial police force, gave us permission to set up a tent and stay. In fact, we were given a choice location: next to the one visible tree on the arid, rolling plain. It was a gnarled, stunted tree with microscopic leaves, but its branches offered the only shade within walking distance of the huts. Our tent proved to be unlivably hot (the Gabra huts were much cooler), so the tree was truly a blessing. Often we would spend the hottest part of the day inching along the dry ground to follow the meager shadows as the earth turned.

There were few insects to bother us. The high winds counteracted the enervation of the heat, and at night the stars were spectacular. From time to time, a hyena or an ostrich would come near the camp, and vultures circled during the day.

On Friday, June 29, when the power of the sun was diminishing in the late afternoon, I sat talking with an elder of the camp who was carving a camel bell out of a piece of wood, and with two younger men. The older man, who said he was sixty, was very thin and had a white beard and an air of nobility. In the past he had served a term as leader of rituals for his section of the tribe. One of the younger men asked me if I knew when the eclipse was going to happen. It was not surprising that these Gabra knew of the eclipse. The Kenyan government had made a great effort to alert all of the populace to it and, in particular, to warn people not to watch it, lest they go blind. These warnings had been disseminated in leaflets, through schools, on radios, and by native policemen.

The Gabra of our camp had doubtless heard of the event at the Maikona well complex.

I replied that the eclipse was due at four in the afternoon. "What do you think will happen?" I asked. The answer surprised me: "We have heard that the government is going to cause the sun to die." I asked whether anyone had ever seen such a thing. The old man said that his great-grandfather had mentioned an eclipse of the sun. "But that was a long time ago; we have never experienced it." He went on to say that his people did have experience of times when the moon "died" and that such times were bad omens, especially for the health of animals. If a lunar eclipse takes place during a certain month of the year it may even signify the impending death of the tribe's ritual leaders. "But as for the sun . . . we don't know. We will have to wait and see."

One of the younger men asked me if I thought they should bring their animals back to camp when the sun died. I said I did not know. The older man asked if the eclipse would hurt your eyes; he had heard that. I told him it was all right to look at the sun when it was black. He then asked if we had camels in America and when I told him no, he asked again, as if he could not imagine a life without camels.

On the morning of the eclipse, Duba invited us to partake of a ritual "sacrifice" of coffee beans in our honor. We had brought some coffee beans and sugar as gifts, and Duba's wife prepared them in the traditional way: We were served wooden goblets of warm camel's milk mixed with a little sugar and camel butter with the whole roasted coffee beans floating on top. It was pleasant to chew the crunchy beans with the sweet liquid; for the Gabra it was a rare treat.

The day was cloudless and warm as usual, and we waited with great anticipation for the partial phase of the eclipse to begin. From time to time I glanced at the sun through a double thickness of exposed film to see if there was any change, but I could detect nothing until about 3:00 P.M., when a visible "bite" appeared in the lower (western) edge of the solar disc. The progress of the partial phase is not very interesting until near the end. In fact, if one glances up with the naked eye (this is harmless for a fraction of a second), the light from the remaining solar disc is still so blinding that one cannot even tell that an eclipse is going on.

I should say at once that I am entirely unable to assess the reaction of the Gabra to the death of the sun. The fact is that the Gabra did not get much chance to watch the eclipse, because shortly before the onset of the partial phase, a three-man film crew from New York arrived in a Land Rover to record their reactions to it. The filmmakers picked this location as the most photogenic in the area and called a hasty meeting with Duba and the other elders to obtain permission to film. Gabra are afraid of being photographed, but with the exchange of a suitable amount of money, Duba agreed to keep his people out of doors during the eclipse and to convince them to be willing subjects. The natural reaction of the people might have been to stay indoors (most of the tribes in the path of totality interpreted the government warnings to mean that they should hide in their dwellings), but the filmmakers had little concern for the fidelity of their "documentary." In fact, to jazz up the proceedings they insisted on building a huge bonfire in front of the huts, around which the willing subjects could be posed in dramatic attitudes.

It was only ten minutes before totality when the firewood for this massive special effect was collected, and the activity of the film crew became feverish, with much running about and shouting orders. The Gabra, who only three days before had lived in peaceful isolation with their camels and thorn-bushes, were now actors on a frenzied movie set complete with cameras, tripods, sound equipment, Land Rover, anthropologist, and assorted white strangers from a part of the world with no camels. To the dismay of the film crew, the bonfire would not light, and an order was given to bring some gasoline. As the driver of the Land Rover ran back with a can of fuel, he tripped and dropped the entire can onto the smoldering woodpile, which exploded in a mushroom of flame that burned the driver, nearly ignited the huts, and sent everyone reeling backward in confusion. The cameras rolled on. To the Gabra these events were far more spectacular (and life-threatening) than the eclipse taking place simultaneously, which is why I say we shall never know how they would have reacted to it alone.

I absented myself from the set as soon as I saw that the fire was under control and concentrated instead on the sky. A cloud cover had come up midway through the partial phase — the heaviest clouds I had seen since coming to the Chalbi — and it seemed for a time that we would be denied a view of the eclipse. But then, miraculously, a hole opened up just around the sun and stayed there. Even before the gasoline explosion, the light had started to change, and I recalled Miahuatlán powerfully. What happens in the last minutes before totality is that the light gets very dim in one way while remaining brilliant in another. In the sky, the slender solar crescent is still too blinding to look at directly, and shadows on the ground are as crisp and dark as on the brightest summer day. But the quality of the light is altogether different — like superbright moonlight. I found myself looking at my hands and arms, at the huts, at the ground, even at the film crew. I wanted to see as much as possible under this novel illumination. It is a living paradox, bright yet dim, like no other light I have ever seen.

And it changes very fast, which adds to the novelty. As the cone of shadow approaches, a sense of drama builds: Something is going to happen. The light fades faster and faster, retaining that curious ghost of solar brightness to the last. Finally, I discarded my exposed film and looked up in time to see the glaring yellow light of the sun reduced to a single point — an effect known to eclipse watchers as the "diamond ring." Then the moon rolled directly in front of the sun, the silvery white corona appeared, and once again I was in the umbra.

*

Immediately after the eclipse, a woman who was part of our group asked how long we had been in the shadow. To her it had seemed like thirty seconds. But someone with a watch had timed it at three and a half minutes. The woman said, "I want more of it." A young man who was with us, as the light was becoming ordinary again, said, "Already it seems like a dream. I remember it exactly the way I remember dreams." Reality inside the umbra is not ordinary reality; the dream-like quality is one manifestation of the difference. Another is the sense of improbability that a still point could exist in the midst of opposing forces. The hurricane's eye must be as improbable: a cylinder of blue sky and sun and calm water in the very center of a system of frenzied energies. In the path of a total eclipse one has the privilege of sharing the perfect alignment of earth, moon, and sun. For a brief interval out of time, the three bodies are frozen in majestic union; then they go on their separate, complicated courses. To participate in that moment of uncanny equilibrium is to have one's faith strengthened in the possibility of equilibrium and to experience the paradox that balance and stillness are to be found at the heart of all change.

Recurrent in the philosophies and myths of peoples around the world are themes of the union of sun and moon, symbolic of the union of conscious and unconscious forces within the human psyche that must take place if one is to become whole. The light of the corona — peaceful, cool, silver-white, normally invisible in the glare of the day — is a perfect representation of the intuitive consciousness that normally is hidden in the glare of ordinary mental activity. It is that hidden consciousness we try to contact by means of meditation, drugs, hypnosis, and other techniques that focus attention or shake us out of ordinary perceptions. And whenever we make that contact — whenever there is an interchange of masculine and feminine energies within our minds — we get high. A total eclipse is one great natural high.

One way to avoid the power of an eclipse is to photograph it. I observed in Africa that the people who spent the precious time of totality taking pictures were visibly less moved by the event than others. In a similar way, scientists who study eclipses shield themselves from the experience by looking at instruments instead of the sky. They cannot possibly be surprised by the appearance of night in day. In Mexico I spent the afternoon before the eclipse at the scientific compound of a major American expedition, watching the astronomers rehearse what they would be doing during totality. They had recorded on tape the sound of a hammer striking an anvil as a monotone voice chanted the elapsed time in seconds. To this unnerving accompaniment, suggestive of the galley of a Roman slave ship, the scientists marched around like robots, their eyes fixed always on their machines. Meanwhile, outside the walled compound, gleeful Mexicans ran about shooting off skyrockets and having the time of their lives in celebration of all the activity that had come to their town. The chief scientist was furious about the rockets. "Can't you stop them?" he kept shouting. "They'll ruin our measurements!" I decided I would be far better able to enjoy the eclipse away from the measurers and chose my hill accordingly.

Scientists and photographers hide from eclipses behind their instruments. Others simply hide — under a cardboard box or in a hut. Several Borana elders told me that the last total eclipse over their land, two generations ago, caught people unawares in open country, where they crouched down and waited until it was over, then appealed to their ritual leaders for interpretation. This time, advised by the government in Nairobi of the danger of blindness due on Saturday, June 30, 1973, at 4:00 P.M., most of the Borana in the path of totality went into their huts when the sun began to "get sick" and could not be coaxed out until the light returned. According to a story in the *East African Standard* of July 2, "Once the sun was more than half covered, most of the women of the Samburu and Turkana tribes moved into their huts, and the less sophisticated El Molo shut themselves up completely in their palm-fronded 'igloos,' placing cardboard or a piece of sacking over the entrance."

The government predicted the eclipse. The eclipse happened. Therefore, the government caused it. And by warning people not to look at it, the Kenyan authorities took advantage of the moon's shadow in order to strengthen their control over the tribes — another step in the transfer of power from local, tribal rule to central, urban rule.

In the memorandum of the Justice Department, nature is

conceived as a hostile trickster, luring us to destruction with "fascinating but dangerous" sights. One might almost think that our government — jealous of powerful events beyond its dominion — also hopes to appropriate eclipses. When events have the potential to get us high by interrupting the ordinary, orderly flow of everyday reality, they are especially threatening to the men in power, who want us to feel threatened along with them. "There is no safe way to view the eclipse directly," says the Justice Department. *"The best way to view the eclipse is on television."* Best for whom?

*

That total eclipses of the sun are threatening to social authorities is clear. Their fear may be justified. Recently, I came across a good historical case that I should forward to the Department of Justice.

In 1890 the last great uprising of the Sioux took place, leading to the massacre at Wounded Knee, South Dakota. The cause of this uprising was the attempt of white Americans to stamp out a new and militant religious movement that appeared suddenly among the mostly defeated Indians. This movement, the Ghost Dance Religion, was part of a messianic wave that swept through the tribes of the West at the end of the 1880s.

The messiah who taught his fellow Indians to dance the Ghost Dance was a Paiute named Wovoka. He lived in Nevada and experienced revelations that drew representatives of many tribes to him. His new religion took hold most firmly among the Sioux, perhaps because their lives had become so hopeless. When Sioux converts followed Wovoka's instructions for the Ghost Dance, they fell on the ground in trances, saw and conversed with dead friends and relatives, experienced a beautiful otherworld, and found new sources of strength and faith. The military authorities were frightened of this development and forbade the Sioux to dance the Ghost Dance.

An article on "The Ghost Dance of 1890" has this to say about the messiah who started it all: "Wovoka seems to

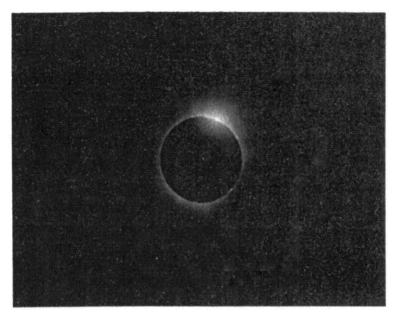

Sun's corona and solar prominences, seen during the total eclipse of February 26, 1979, at Brandon, Manitoba, Canada. (Jay Pasachoff)

have had his first revelation in about 1887, after which he began to teach the dance to his people. His most important vision, however, came on January 1, 1889, in conjunction with a total eclipse of the sun. On this occasion he felt himself to be taken up into the spirit world, where he met the supernatural and was given a message to convey to his people." *

*

With each recent eclipse, authorities have been more and more successful in persuading the general populace to share their fears. The total eclipse of February 26, 1979, evoked behavior in Canada that I found incomprehensible. I traveled to southern Manitoba for the event and viewed it from a snow-covered field near the town of Brandon in subfreezing weather.

* Thomas W. Overholt, *Ethnohistory* 21, No. 1 (Winter 1974): 41.

That eclipse was billed as the last total eclipse of the sun visible from the United States and Canada in the twentieth century, which might be fortunate, considering how most people reacted to it. The path of totality included Winnipeg, the capital of Manitoba, a city of half a million inhabitants.

In December 1978 the city Health Department wrote the Manitoba Medical Association asking advice on what to do about the eclipse. The association replied in a letter dated January 10, 1979:

> The Section of Ophthalmology of the Manitoba Medical Association strongly advises that the only safe method of viewing the sun, especially in eclipse, is to watch it on television. No other means is completely reliable . . . Nothing short of 100 percent foolproof protection is called for when the stakes are as high as permanent loss of vision. Again, the M.M.A. Section of Ophthalmology advises that the eclipse of the sun should only be viewed on television. This position is also endorsed by the Canadian Ophthalmological Society.

In response to this alarm, the Health Department notified the superintendent of schools of the danger. Totality in Winnipeg was due at 11:46 on a Monday morning. Normally, schoolchildren would be dismissed at 11:30 for lunch. In mid-January the school superintendent sent a memorandum to all school principals laying down guidelines for eclipse day. These included the following steps:

> (1) . . . care must be taken to have all students indoors before the eclipse begins; (2) arrangements will have to be made to keep students in school until about 12:05 P.M.; (3) blinds and/or drapes will have to be lowered or drawn over windows facing the sun to prevent accidental exposure during the eclipse; (4) all staff have the responsibility of doing their utmost to protect students at school from possible injury, according to the advice given to us by the City of Winnipeg Health Department and the Manitoba Medical Association.

A week before the eclipse, the superintendent sent out another memorandum with further specifications, including plans to prevent children from playing hookey, sneaking off to washrooms, or otherwise trying to get a glimpse of the sky that morning. It concluded: "I am sure by now you are hoping for a cloudy day. We have responsibilities both from a health point of view and a legal point of view, and I am trying to follow the best advice we can get in order to safeguard both."

The ultimate absurdity came a few days later in a memorandum concerning the possibility of fire alarms sounding during the eclipse. It began: "When the alarm sounds the classes will remain in their locations or rooms and await further instructions." One suspected that the school board would almost prefer to see its charges burn to death than have any exposure to the malevolent rays of the eclipsed sun.

Despite the efforts of some thoughtful persons, especially astronomers, this irrational phobia prevailed. Winnipeg schoolchildren were denied the glorious sight of the eclipse. Many families huddled by their television sets with blankets hung over their windows. Radio announcers warned that "a moment's reckless pleasure was hardly worth a lifetime of misery and blindness." Moreover, those who joined in this collective madness congratulated themselves on being informed, scientific, and civilized.

Naturally, those who just looked up at the sky were awed. A small victory, in fact, was that the Canadian Broadcasting Commission radio announcer, perched on the roof of a Winnipeg office building, was struck dumb by the beauty of the eclipse and remained silent for some of the period of totality.

I would like to know the origin of this unhealthy fear. Older people remember nothing of the sort at eclipses in the early part of this century. In an old *National Geographic* there is a photograph of President Hoover casually viewing the solar eclipse of 1932 from the White House lawn, using a piece of exposed film. In Washington that eclipse was only 89 percent total. On the facing page, crowds of people are shown viewing the same eclipse from the top of the Empire State Building in New York City, again using only exposed film.

Solar eclipse phobia is a product of recent times. I am

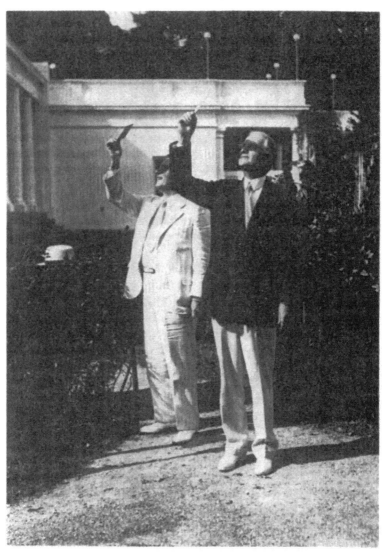

President Hoover views the solar eclipse of August 31, 1932, from the White House grounds. The path of totality of this eclipse crossed New Hampshire and Maine. In Washington, a partial eclipse of 89 percent totality occurred. Partial eclipses are more dangerous to observe than full eclipses because the sun is not completely covered. Mr. Hoover appears to be using nothing more than a piece of exposed film, yet history does not record that he went blind in 1932 or anytime thereafter. (Historical Pictures Service)

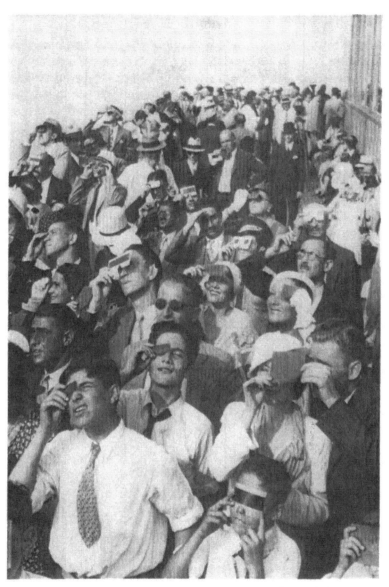

Hundreds of people gathered on the observation platform of the Empire State Building in New York City to view the eclipse of August 31, 1932. There, too, the eclipse was almost total but not quite. In this more innocent age, fears of blindness did not keep people from watching the moon cover the sun. (Wide World Photos)

afraid it is a measure of how much our technological society has alienated us from nature and how much our technological medicine has become a kind of state religion. It is doctors who provide the rationale for hiding with our television sets behind blanketed windows and denying ourselves one of the great highs of nature. It is all of us who let them get away with it.

19

THE MARRIAGE OF THE
SUN AND MOON

MANY WRITERS on consciousness have pointed out that states very real to those who experience them are frequently difficult to describe or document objectively. As a consequence, a great discrepancy exists between direct, experiential knowledge of altered states of awareness and theoretical understanding of them. And because individuals in our culture do not readily discuss their experiences of this sort, even the experiential knowledge does not circulate freely.

I must emphasize at the outset my prejudice that the experience of an altered state of consciousness is intrinsically more valuable than any amount of theorizing about it, unless the theory helps individuals to make more and better use of the states available to them.

Several years ago I published a comprehensive theory of altered states of consciousness based primarily on personal experience and secondarily on objective experiment and observation.* (It is worth remembering that the words *experience* and *experiment* come from the same root.) The main points of that theory were the following:

- Human beings are born with a drive to experience modes of awareness other than the normal waking one; from very young ages, children experiment with techniques to change consciousness.

* Andrew Weil, *The Natural Mind: A New Way of Looking at Drugs and the Higher Consciousness* (Boston: Houghton Mifflin, 1972).

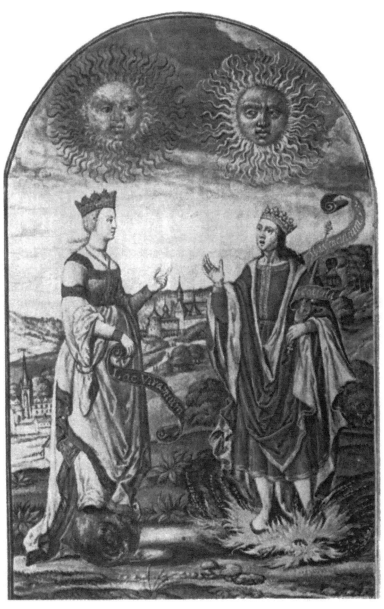

Coniunctio solis et lunae. One version of the alchemical theme of the marriage of the sun and moon, this from "Splendor solis" by Salomon Trismo-
sin, a manuscript from 1582.

- Such experiences are normal. Every person spends large amounts of time in other states, whether he or she retains awareness of them or not.
- Altered states of consciousness form a continuous spectrum from ordinary waking consciousness. For example, there is no qualitative difference between watching a movie (light concentration) and being in a trance (deep concentration).
- Although specific external triggers, such as drugs, may elicit these states, they do not cause them. Alternate states of consciousness arise from interactions among purely intrapsychic forces. External triggers provide opportunities for people to allow themselves certain experiences that may also be had without the triggers. Thus, a drug-induced state may be essentially the same as one induced by chanting or meditating.
- It is valuable to learn to enter other states deliberately and consciously because such experiences are doorways to fuller use of the nervous system, to the realization of untapped human potential, and to better functioning in the ordinary mode of consciousness.

*

People in the path of a total eclipse of the sun experience dramatic alterations in consciousness if they allow themselves to view the event. As explained in the previous chapter, surprisingly many people who are overtaken by eclipses do not watch them because they are afraid. In primitive societies eclipses signify bad luck of one sort or another. In civilized societies the same attitude crops up as an irrational fear of blindness. Those who overcome their fears and look directly at total eclipses experience derealization, changes in time perception, and dreamlike feelings of detachment from the external world. Immediately after an eclipse, euphoria is pronounced among those who have watched, and many people continue to feel high and energetic for hours.

Why does a total eclipse of the sun make people high? Possibly the novel light of the corona shakes us out of our usual perceptual framework, enabling us to see our relationship to external reality in a new way. Possibly the exact alignment of earth, moon, and sun has some special and direct effect on brain function. I am afraid that any suggested explanation must be the purest guesswork. There is simply no information about the influence of eclipses on consciousness. In fact, there is no recognition in the literature on altered states that eclipses are one pathway to them.

In the light of my eclipse experiences I find it most interesting that the esoteric traditions of both the East and the West use images of the conjunction of the sun and the moon to convey information about the potential of the mind. In European alchemy, for example, the "marriage of the sun and moon" is a symbolic description of the work to be accomplished. A similar image is the compounding of gold and silver, the metals that stand for the same principles as the two heavenly bodies. Esoteric alchemy was not merely an exercise of physical transformations of material elements but, more important, a set of coded instructions for self-development that could lead eventually to the gold of enlightenment. Yogic literature talks about electric (solar) and magnetic (lunar) nerve currents in the human body and the need for harmonizing and blending the two. These conceptualizations all point to the existence of two distinct aspects of mind that stand in relation to each other as the sun and moon in the sky. Moreover, the suggestion is clear that the psychological basis of high states is an interchange of energies between the solar and lunar compartments of the mind.

Nearly all commentators have recognized a fundamental dualism in the mind and have relegated different types of mental events to one of two opposite and complementary psychic spaces. There are many names for these two compartments,* but there is also high consistency from system to system about their characteristics. That aspect of mind most active in ordinary waking consciousness, which uses intellect as the chief means of making sense of reality and manipulates verbal symbols, is often seen as masculine,

* Robert Ornstein, *The Psychology of Consciousness* (San Francisco: Freeman, 1972), pp. 64–67; Arthur J. Deikman, "Bimodal Consciousness," *Archives of General Psychiatry* 25 (1971): 481–89.

right-handed (in the symbolic sense), and day-oriented. Complementing it and contrasting with it is the feminine, left-handed, nighttime consciousness: the realm of dreams, intuitions, and nonverbal communication.

It is difficult to find neutral names for these two phases of human consciousness because each set is the property of one special-interest group or another. In the past I have used the terms *conscious* and *unconscious*, but these have particular meanings in psychoanalytic theory, a model I do not find useful in trying to understand other states of consciousness. Furthermore, I no longer believe in the aptness of the word *unconscious* to describe the night side of the mind. In the symbolism of the Tarot cards, day consciousness is represented by the Magician, a male figure standing in a gesture of active concentration; he is associated with the color yellow. His complement is the High Priestess, a blue-robed virgin, seated in a receptive pose. These symbols, in their details, are good depictions of the nature and potential of the two phases of mind, but they are part of a larger collection of symbols irrelevant to the present discussion.

Perhaps the most neutral of the symbols available to us are the primal representations of the basic dualism of reality: the sun and the moon. Not only are these heavenly bodies familiar to all of us, they have struck many thinkers as appropriate designations for the masculine and feminine aspects of human consciousness. The moon, especially, represents well the night side of the mind. Indeed, the High Priestess of the Tarot deck is nothing other than the virgin moon goddess who appears in the celestial hierarchies of so many cultures.

I propose, then, to use the terms *solar* and *lunar* to denote the two compartments of human mental activity. Although I am not suggesting any causal relationships between the sun and moon and mental events, I do believe in a tight correlation between the qualities of those bodies and the qualities of the two phases of consciousness. In particular, I would draw attention to the sun's property of overwhelming all other sources of light and radiation when it is above the horizon and the moon's cyclic waxing and waning in intensity. The sun and the moon are symbolic of the mind in the true sense of the word; that is, they not only represent the dualism of consciousness but are actually expressions of that same dualism, which is manifest in the sky as well as the mind. This is an important point: After all, the actual union of the sun and the moon during the moments of a total eclipse does, in fact, make people high.

If the psychological basis of altered states is some sort of interchange of energies between the solar mind and the lunar mind, what, then, is the situation in ordinary waking awareness? It seems reasonable to compare ordinary consciousness to ordinary daytime. The sun shines in the sky, and the moon is invisible. Many people in our society never see much of the moon. They live in cities, where buildings and artificial light hinder observation of the night sky, and they are indoors or asleep while the moon passes through its cycle. Reasoning by analogy, we may conclude that many people in our society are also relatively unconscious of the lunar forces within themselves. Possibly, the tendency to describe the lunar mind as unconscious indicates how commonly we deny it access to the ordinarily conscious solar mind.

Presumably, two distinct kinds of changes would alter the ordinary condition of the mind. Anything that diminished or focused the intensity of the solar mind might enable it to notice, and interact more with, the lunar mind. Anything that stimulated the lunar mind might permit it to achieve balance and interact with the solar mind. Various methods of achieving high states of consciousness illustrate these complementary approaches.

*

Many kinds of mushrooms are capable of triggering altered states of consciousness. Throughout the world, human cultures have linked mushrooms with the moon and with water, the feminine or lunar element, as opposed to fire, which is masculine and solar. In chapters 7–9 I wrote that mushrooms are powerful symbols of lunar forces, meaning that they actually embody those forces and do not simply represent them. Mushrooms are associated also with death and madness (lunacy), with flights of the soul from the body, with night and magic — in short, with many manifestations of the realm of experience that is normally unconscious in most of us.

People who eat psychoactive mushrooms often remain very aware of the taste of the fungus during the intoxication. Some users feel that taste diffused throughout their bodies. Many people report visions of mushrooms. Regular users interpret these sensory experiences as indications of the flooding of their bodies and minds with some kind of energy peculiar to mushrooms. I think mushrooms do give us high doses of lunar or yin energy. Furthermore, I think it is reasonable to propose that mushrooms stimulate the lunar sphere of the mind, causing changes in consciousness by intensifying the activity of that sphere so that it comes more into balance with the solar mind.

Here, perhaps, is an explanation of mycophobia — fear of mushrooms — which is so prevalent among human beings. Mycophobia is vastly out of proportion to the actual risk of serious mushroom poisoning. I would guess that it really reflects fear of the darker side of the human mind, that it originates in the solar sphere, and that it is a manifestation of the same uneasiness that expresses itself as fear and ambivalence about drugs, eclipses, and other external objects and events that bring about changes in consciousness by establishing new relationships between the two compartments of the mind.

*

Sweat bathing is a common ritual among North American Indians. It is both a hygienic practice and a religious one. As a religious ritual, it is an intense experience that produces marked alterations in consciousness.

The sweat lodge is of simple construction: an open framework of willow saplings bent and tied together to form a

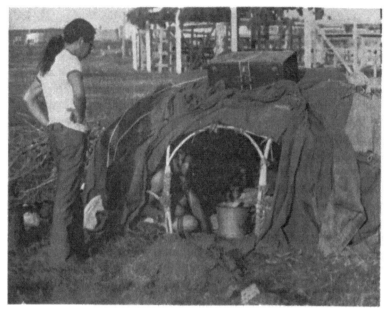

A Sioux sweat lodge ready for use. (Thomas E. Mails)

circular hut perhaps five feet in diameter and three or four feet high. Over this framework are draped animal hides, canvas, or blankets so that the interior is completely dark and insulated. A shallow pit is dug in the earth in the center of the lodge. Participants in the ritual, usually from four to eight depending on the size of the lodge, sit unclothed on the ground. Attendants on the outside fill the pit with red-hot rocks that have been heated in a strong bonfire. The lodge is then sealed up from outside, leaving the participants in darkness and increasing heat.

Among the Sioux, the sweat lodge is consecrated ground on which man contacts the Great Spirit of the Universe. Sprigs of sage are placed among the willow poles, and cedar incense is burned on the hot rocks as the ritual begins. The medicine man in charge of the sweat offers prayers for the efficacy of the ritual and for the safety of the participants. He passes around the sacred pipe filled with an aromatic mixture of tobacco and red-willow bark. Each person prays

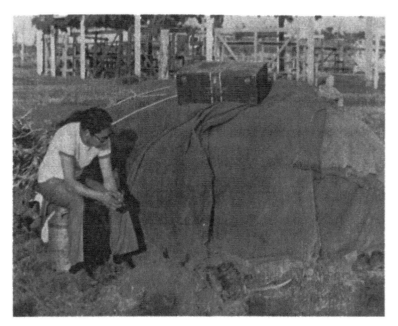

The Sioux sweat lodge in operation. (Thomas E. Mails)

with the pipe and smokes it. The leader then begins his chants. When he is finished he starts to throw water on the glowing rocks.

As the water hits the rocks, an explosive hiss seems to shake the lodge. Seconds later a wave of intense heat envelops the body. As soon as this wave passes, the leader adds more water, causing another explosion of sound in the darkness and another wave of intense sensation, stronger than the last. The process continues until no one can stand any more, at which point the shouting of a special phrase (meaning "All my relations!") signals the outside attendants to throw off the coverings of the lodge, leaving it open to the winds. As soon as the participants recover, the lodge is sealed again, and another cycle of praying, smoking, chanting, and scalding takes place. A full ceremony may include four or five cycles of increasing intensity.

When the sweat lodge is used simply to clean the body of surface dirt or to warm the bones in a cold climate, it offers a pleasant experience but one that does not transcend the ordinary. However, when a powerful medicine man conducts a solemn ritual therein, the sweat lodge can provide a life-changing experience.

I was introduced to the sweat lodge by a Sioux medicine man on the Rosebud Reservation in South Dakota. The first time I was in the lodge I could not believe how hot it got. The sensation of live steam was so strong that I thought my skin was on fire, and I quickly learned that I had to keep wiping the sweat off my skin to avoid getting burned. (Water conducts heat to the skin faster than air.) It is possible to get first- or second-degree burns in the sweat lodge, but, curiously enough, one's mental state seems to be the most important determinant of the fate of one's skin. Burning occurs only when you lose contact with the psychic energy of the group and see yourself as an isolated individual trying to defend yourself against the onslaught of heat. With trust and confidence in the medicine man and willingness to abandon yourself to the powers in the sweat lodge, you do not suffer physical damage, even though the sensations are as intense as any you have ever felt and the temperature in the lodge is near 212°F (100°C) for brief periods.

In the sweat lodge one meets and conquers many fears. All the terrors of darkness, noise, fire, and helplessness rise up to challenge the participants in the ritual and are defeated by the collective faith of the group. When the steam explodes from the rocks there is no time for thinking; all mental effort is focused on the wave of heat about to break. Coping with that wave, receiving it, and riding over its crest take full concentration. The reward of perseverance is a terrific high. At the end of a good sweat, people feel euphoric, lifted out of themselves, purged of anxiety and depression, healthy, and full of energy. On coming out of sweat lodges, I have felt high in many of the same ways I have felt on using psychedelic drugs. The high lasts an hour or so and gradually gives way to great relaxation and a desire to rest. Increased awareness of one's own strength and a sense of well-being may persist for a long time.

The devices by which the sweat lodge brings about a high seem to me to operate on the solar compartment of the mind. The act of entering the darkness of the lodge in the first place is a symbolic withdrawal from the ordinary world of daylight. The chanting of the medicine man brings about an initial degree of concentration, the prerequisite for many kinds of altered states. Chanting, whatever its form, is a powerful technique to change consciousness. It seems to work by occupying the ordinary mind that is usually busy thinking and paying attention to multifarious external stimuli. In a similar way, the sharp noise of the steam focuses awareness on a specific auditory sensation, increasing the depth of concentration. But it is the intense waves of heat that carry this process to an unusual extreme. There is no question that the experience in the sweat lodge would be horribly painful to someone unprepared for it. Nor is there anything unusual about pain serving as the basis for alterations of consciousness. What is interesting about the sweat lodge is that set and setting encourage the participants to interpret the strong stimulation as good and healthy and that with this set and setting the sensation is one of pain that does not hurt. And what is more, this experience of pain that does not hurt leads to a powerful high in the complete absence of tissue injury.

Nonhurtful pain is well known in hypnosis and other trance states and with the administration of opiates. It is less well known in psychedelic states, but I have seen it occur there often, again leading to highs. Now, it is important to distinguish between the anesthesia of hysterical dissociation and the high experience of nonhurtful pain. A badly wounded soldier on a battlefield may perform heroically, unaware of his injuries. A mother, seeing her child pinned beneath a car, may lift the car unassisted and be unaware that she has suffered crushing fractures of her vertebrae until she learns that the child is all right. In these cases, intense emotion leads to a kind of trance state in which a barrier develops between nerve impulses from the body and awareness centers in the higher brain. Real injury has occurred, but the message of it does not make it through to consciousness for some time. By contrast, in the experience of nonhurtful pain, full awareness of the body persists. Sensations are perceived as strong but not noxious; no injury results; and one feels energetic and high at the end. It is tempting to invoke something like hysterical dissociation to explain this experience, but that mechanism, although it can account for anesthesia, cannot explain the absence of tissue injury despite stimulation that would certainly cause damage under other circumstances.

I had my first experience of nonhurtful pain under the influence of LSD. I found myself walking barefoot over a stretch of sharp stones near my house that I had never been able to walk on before. I was very aware of the pressure of the stones on my feet, but the sensation was simply strong and neutral. This feeling was so novel that I explored it for some time, running back and forth on the stones and jumping up and down on them. Yet at the end of this experience I had not the slightest marks on the soles of my feet. A few days later, when feeling ordinary, I tried to walk over the stones again but could not repeat my performance. Even a few steps hurt and left marks.

The Sioux sweat lodge, without psychedelics, reinforced my belief in the importance of the phenomenon of nonhurtful pain and motivated me to experiment further. Using LSD and MDA, I found that under certain circumstances I could interact with fire or hot or sharp objects or receive strong blows on the body but suffer no injury. A high followed from the interaction. The drugs did not automatically confer this immunity from damaging pain but simply made the experience more likely; I still had to be in the right frame of mind. After a number of practice sessions, I found that I could reproduce the experience without drugs, especially if I was with others who had had such experiences and we used chanting as a means of producing the necessary state of concentration. I discern the following principles at work in this process:

There is a psychophysical state in which powerful sensations that would normally be perceived as painful and cause bodily damage do not hurt and do cause highs.

Fear of the stimulus is the greatest obstacle to this experience.

The presence of someone who has experienced the state and is not afraid of the stimulus is the greatest facilitator of the experience.

A preliminary degree of concentration is necessary for the state to occur. Chanting, drugs, hypnosis, and probably many other techniques can bring about such concentration.

Concentration is greatly deepened by the stimulus itself. During the experience of nonhurtful pain, all attention is on the sensations coming from the body, with none on verbal thought. In other words, the activity of the solar mind is highly focused.

The high of this state begins during the period of intense stimulation and reaches a maximum after the stimulation ends.

I would like to offer a hypothetical mechanism to explain the experience of pain that does not hurt. A strong stimulus presents the body with a challenge of energy: thermal energy in the case of steam or fire, kinetic energy in the case of a blow. How the body deals with this energy depends on the state of the nervous system when the stimulus arrives. Under certain conditions the peripheral nervous system might be capable of receiving unusually large amounts of physical energy, transmuting them electrochemically, and conducting them away from the periphery to the central nervous system. In the central nervous system, this energy could be discharged through the head in some harmless way or experienced as a high. The peripheral tissues, meanwhile, would be spared any adverse effects.

Such receptivity of the peripheral nervous system could occur only in the absence of interference from the higher mind. A state of fear or an effort to defend oneself against the perceived threat of strong stimulation might create a condition of neuromuscular tension that would impair or prevent peripheral nervous receptivity. The energy of the stimulus would then not be able to flow into the nerves directly but would instead spill into the peripheral tissues, causing damage and pain. The experience of pain would then increase neuromuscular tension in a vicious cycle.

In this scheme, the hypothesized condition of peripheral nervous receptivity would be a consequence of a particular central state. Specifically, a balanced interchange of energy between the solar and lunar compartments of the mind would permit the central nervous system to enter into the necessary relationship with the peripheral. This interchange might arise through stimulation of the lunar compartment or focusing of the solar compartment, or both.

My interest in the potential of the human nervous system to interact with unusually strong forces has led me to review the literature on fire walking as practiced throughout much of Asia and in some Western countries, such as Greece. There is much documentation, both written and photographic, of the ability of human beings, under certain circumstances, to walk unprotected on red-hot coals or stones or through bonfires.* There has been little scientific study of fire walking, and generally scientists have sought materialistic explanations of the phenomenon. Some have proposed, not very imaginatively, that Asians have tougher feet than non-Asians or that fire walkers are simply deceiving Western observers in one way or another. Others have suggested that perspiration forms a thin insulating layer that protects the skin from the heat.

My personal experiences with the sweat lodge make me less inclined to look for simple physical explanations of fire walking. I note that the presence of experienced fire walkers is necessary for the success of novices. Usually, participants in fire walking rituals work themselves up to the main events by long periods of chanting and dancing. Among certain Hindu fire walkers of Singapore, whipping is used to banish fear and deepen concentration. Apparently, the blows

---

* Richard P. Leavitt in *New York Times*, April 29, 1973; Victor Perera, "Foreign Notes: The Firewalkers of Upappawa," *Harper's*, May 1971, pp. 18–21.

cause no pain or injury, although they are delivered with great force.* Certain Japanese Buddhist sects perform ritual walks over red-hot coals while chanting silently a particular sutra. I have interviewed several members of one of these sects. They confirm the suppositions that concentration is vital, that a break in concentration (in this case in the rhythm of the chant) leads to burns, and that successful completion of the fire walk results in a powerful high, marked by euphoria, energy, and new confidence in one's abilities and strengths. All of this leads me to conclude that the true explanation of the ability to walk through fire unharmed lies in a different functioning of the nervous system brought about by a change in relationship between the solar and lunar compartments of the mind.

*

The greatest difficulty in the scientific study of consciousness today is the gulf between materialistic and nonmaterialistic views of the mind. It is unfortunately true that most neuroscientists are hard-core materialists who cannot believe in the reality of experiences without obvious physical bases. Because we are far from understanding the physical mechanisms of altered states of consciousness, many scientists who study the brain are able to dismiss the whole field as mystical nonsense. A neurochemist investigating dopamine receptors in the limbic forebrain would have little time for the concept of a solar and a lunar mind that I have used in this chapter, even though the limbic forebrain may turn out to be an important locus of lunar consciousness.

A complementary problem exists with psychiatrists and psychologists who use abstract concepts like id and ego but resist the idea that such concepts must correlate with physiological realities. The early Freudians ostracized Wilhelm Reich chiefly because he insisted that unconscious experiences were recorded in the muscles and could be reached by

* A. Babb, "Walking on Flowers in Singapore: A Hindu Festival Cycle," Working Paper No. 27 of the Department of Sociology, University of Singapore, 1974 (unpublished manuscript).

manipulation of the body as well as the mind. Modern Freudians still are uncomfortable with suggestions that the unconscious is anything but an abstraction. For example, psychoanalysts regard the dream world as essentially unreal, full of symbols to be used in the analytic process but certainly not an actual place available for visiting. Psychoanalysts cannot make sense of the process of dream yoga as practiced by some Tibetan Buddhists and the Senoi people of Malaysia* and as taught by don Juan to Carlos Castaneda,† in which the dreamer learns to enter the dream world consciously and eventually to manipulate it. A cornerstone of the present theory of altered states is that the lunar sphere of the mind is as real as the solar, connected with the activity of real parts of the real brain, unconscious only because we live mostly in our solar minds and direct most of our waking attention there.

If we are to make headway, we must find areas of contact between experiential knowledge of other states and experimental knowledge of the nervous system. Of course, some such efforts are under way. In the past few years, for example, there has been much talk of differential functioning of the left and right cerebral hemispheres. Some people would like to equate this anatomical division with the dualism in mind seen by most psychologists interested in consciousness. In providing common ground on which neuroscientists and psychologists may meet, this work has done a good service. But I am not sure it points us in the right direction.

Although a difference certainly exists between the two hemispheres, particularly in regard to language, I do not believe the two sides of consciousness can be equated with the two halves of the brain. The mistake comes of interpreting too literally the distinction between left and right. The

* Kilton Stewart, "Dream Theory in Malaya," in *Altered States of Consciousness*, ed. C. T. Tart (Garden City, New York: Anchor Books, 1974), pp. 161–70.

† Carlos Castaneda, *Journey to Ixtlan: The Lessons of Don Juan* (New York: Simon and Schuster, 1972), 126–29.

most extreme version of this mistake I have encountered is a system of mind development recommended in certain southern California circles. It consists of binding the right arm in a cast and sling in order to develop the nondominant cerebral hemisphere and thereby the intuitive faculties. *Left* and *right* should be construed as symbolic designations of the two phases of mind. I believe we can correlate these two aspects of consciousness with different brain loci but that we are much more likely to have success in looking for a vertical split than a horizontal one. *Left* to me connotes below and within as opposed to above and without. Thus, I see the natural locus of lunar consciousness as deep-brain and brainstem structures as opposed to cortical ones, and I am hopeful that one day we will be able to detect increased activity of the deep centers during experiences of alternate states.

As a physician, I am acutely aware of the widespread ignorance of high states in my profession, a situation most unfortunate in view of the tremendous implications of these states for medicine. For years, psychiatrists in the Freudian tradition and doctors who look to them for authoritative concepts have dismissed certain common powerful experiences as "oceanic feelings" of no great significance. I am convinced that it is during such episodes that the nervous system is in the special physiological state I have described as the basis of the experience of nonhurtful pain. Very few physicians and psychiatrists know the reality of that experience or its vast significance. Not only is it a natural high of great personal worth and meaning; it also represents a condition of unity between mind and body that may be supremely valuable and logical, appearing unusual only because we have been conditioned to believe that such unity is impossible.

It is the intimate connection between the experience of being high and the dramatic change in physiological response to the environment that leads me to see great evolutionary logic in the strong tendency of human beings to search for ways of changing consciousness. I have written elsewhere about activities of young children that serve to alter consciousness * and have suggested that these activities are universally present in human cultures, representing an innate drive arising from the structure of the human nervous system. I include such behaviors as the rhythmic rocking of infants who have just learned to sit up, the spinning and whirling of older children, and games of hyperventilation and mutual choking or chest squeezing. I continue to regard these activities as very widespread if not ubiquitous and am amazed that a number of psychiatrists, including some child psychiatrists, have stated publicly that they have never seen children engage in them. Of course, children do not perform these behaviors in the offices of psychiatrists and often keep this sort of play secret from grownups. Recently, a colleague of mine who is in grade school administered a questionnaire about spinning to her classmates and to other schoolchildren. A very high percentage of respondents admitted to being spinners, and some were quite eloquent as to what they liked about the activity. Here are the statements of some ten-year-olds: "It gets you dizzy and it makes you feel good." "It's like you've gone crazy." "It's like I'm flying." "I like the floating feeling." "I feel energy going around my body." "It's just fun." Clearly, these children are experiencing changes in consciousness.

I hope it will be possible to gather more statistical data on the occurrence of these behaviors and to look for correlations with other variables. Are the children who spin better daydreamers? Will they as adults be most likely to experiment with psychoactive drugs? Are they more creative than nonspinners? It would be interesting and useful to know the answers to these questions.

We live in an age favorable to the investigation of our subject. In many past ages, manifestations of lunar consciousness were regarded as nonexistent or evil. People who tried to draw attention to their reality and importance were shouted down or driven out of respectable intellectual cir-

---

* Weil, *The Natural Mind*, p. 20.

cles. Today, there is increasing acceptance of the lunar side of human nature and the beginnings of willingness to try to integrate that half of consciousness with the solar. This process is not without its dangers. The lunar sphere, though it is a place of great power and the doorway to full realization of the potential of the nervous system, must not be allowed to overwhelm the solar mind. The lunar world is also the world of illusion, chaos, and madness. For just that reason, our ordinary minds prefer not to have much to do with it. Denied the modifying influence of lunar activity, our ordinary minds are sterile; without the directing and guiding function of solar consciousness, the lunar mind is productive of disorder, violence, and insanity.

When people who have lived exclusively in ordinary consciousness begin to contact the mind that is below and within, whether by drugs or meditation or the yoga of dreams or whatever, they may tend to reject rational intellect and other functions of the solar mind in favor of the visions they discover. It is important for students of consciousness, in their own lives and in their work, to demonstrate that the goal is to open the channels between the two minds and to encourage back-and-forth flow between the two without stifling either one. In this way we can become truly whole and healthy and begin to see that the distinctions we have made between mind and body, self and not-self, man and nature, are merely external projections of an unnatural separation we have come to accept within ourselves.

GLOSSARY
SUGGESTED READING
INDEX

GLOSSARY

Accommodation — Process by which certain muscles change the shape of the lens of the eye to allow us to focus on objects at different distances.

Addiction — In reference to drugs, a pattern of consumption marked by compulsive taking of a drug, the need for increasing doses over time to maintain the same effect (tolerance), and the appearance of symptoms when the drug is stopped that disappear when it is reinstituted (withdrawal).

Alcoholic gastritis — Inflammation of the lining of the stomach due to excessive consumption of alcohol.

Alkali — Opposite of acid. Any substance that in solution gives a pH of greater than 7.0. Lye (potassium or sodium hydroxide), baking soda (sodium bicarbonate), and lime (calcium oxide or calcium hydroxide) are examples of alkalies.

Alkaloid — A substance of plant origin, containing nitrogen, that gives a feeble alkaline reaction in solution. Many alkaloids cause pharmacological effects in animals. Their names end in "-ine." Caffeine, morphine, quinine, and nicotine are examples of alkaloids.

Allopathy — Orthodox or "scientific" medicine. A name coined by Samuel Hahnemann to distinguish regular medicine from his new system of homeopathy. (See Homeopath.)

Altered states of consciousness — The spectrum of experiences other than ordinary waking consciousness, including daydreaming, trance, meditation, hypnosis, religious ecstasy, and so forth. Drug-induced highs are varieties of altered states of consciousness.

Amanita — A large genus of gilled mushrooms, distinguished by white gills and spores, a ring around the stipe (called an annulus or partial veil) and a cup at the base of the stipe (the volva). Some amanitas are deadly poisonous.

Ambivalence — A word coined by Freud to indicate the simultaneous existence of conflicting thoughts or feelings, such as love and hate.

Anthurium — A genus of tropical plants in the Jack-in-the-pulpit family, native to Colombia and widely cultivated for their beautiful flowering structures, which consist of a shiny, waxy spathe, often red, and a yellow, fingerlike spadix.

Antispasmodic — A drug that counteracts spasm, relaxing muscular organs.

Astringent — Causing tissues to draw together or contract.

Atropine — An alkaloid found in many plants of the nightshade family that blocks nerve impulses in the parasympathetic nervous system (q.v.). It is used in medicine as an antidote for nerve gas poisoning, as a treatment for gastrointestinal spasm, and as a presurgical drug to dry secretions in the respiratory tract.

Autonomic nervous system — That part of the nervous system regulating involuntary action, as of the heart, glands, and intestines.

Belladonna — The Deadly Nightshade, *Atropa belladonna*, a source of atropine (q.v.). The name means "beautiful lady," because Italian women of the Middle Ages were supposed to have put drops of it in their eyes to make themselves more attractive by dilating their pupils.

"Blow" — Slang term for cocaine.

Brainstem — A group of structures connecting the cerebral hemispheres with the spinal cord. From top to bottom they are: the thalamus (or diencephalon), midbrain, pons, and medulla oblongata.

Cacao — *Theobroma cacao*, a tropical tree, source of cacao beans. The beans contain a high proportion of fat, called cocoa butter. If the beans are heated, ground to a paste, and enriched with additional cocoa butter, the product is chocolate. Ground, defatted beans make cocoa. White chocolate is cocoa butter mixed with sugar.

Central nervous system — The brain and spinal cord.

Centrifugation — The process of spinning a mixture of substances in a machine called a centrifuge in order to separate components of different densities.

Chiropractor — Practitioner of a system of manipulation of the spine to treat disease. Chiropractic was invented by an Iowa grocer, Daniel David Palmer, in 1895. The word means "done by hand."

Conscious mind — That part of the mind characterized by self-awareness.

Cordillera (Spanish) — A major chain of mountains, like the Andes in South America.

Cortex — (Literally "rind.") Referring to the brain, the outer layer of gray matter covering the cerebral hemispheres. It is presumably the seat of higher mental functions, such as thinking, intellect, volition, and so forth.

Decoction — Preparation of a medicinal plant made by boiling the material in water, as opposed to an infusion, in which the substance is merely steeped. Infusions are appropriate for leaves and flowers. Woods, barks, and roots are often prepared as decoctions.

Dopamine — A simple chemical believed to act as a neurotransmitter in parts of the brain by serving as a messenger between one nerve and another.

Drug — A substance that in small doses produces alterations in the body or mind, or both. The decision to call some things drugs and others not is sometimes arbitrary. Salt may function as a drug, yet we think of it as a seasoning or nutrient.

ESP — Extrasensory perception. Acquisition of information through channels other than the five senses. Sometimes used as a synonym for telepathy or mind-to-mind transmission of information.

Fungus — Any of numerous organisms that lack chlorophyll and reproduce by spores, ranging in form from a single cell to a mass of branched filaments that may produce specialized fruiting bodies. Yeasts, molds, rusts, smuts, and mushrooms are all examples.

Henbane — *Hyoscyamus niger*, a psychoactive and toxic plant of the nightshade family, containing the tropane alkaloids (q.v.), used in European witchcraft of the Middle Ages.

High — An altered state of consciousness marked by euphoria, feelings of lightness, self-transcendence, and energy. High states are not necessarily drug-related. They may occur spontaneously or in response to various activities that affect mood, perception, and concentration.

Homeopath — A medical practitioner who follows the precepts of Samuel Hahnemann (1755–1843), the German physician who invented homeopathy. Homeopaths believe that people get sick in unique ways and that they can be cured by administering minute doses of substances that, given in large doses to healthy persons, would reproduce the unique pattern of symptoms. Homeopathy was very strong in Europe and America in the mid-nineteenth century, declined with the rise of technological medicine, and now is having a modest resurgence.

Hyoscyamine — One of the tropane alkaloids, found in many plants of the nightshade family, named for *Hyoscyamus niger*, or Henbane. Like atropine, it blocks neurotransmission in the parasympathetic nervous system.

Hysterical dissociation — An abnormal separation of the conscious, observing mind from other areas of mental function, often occurring under severe stress. In dissociative states, people may perform complicated actions automatically and unconsciously, being oblivious to pain or injury they may have suffered. In lay terminology this condition is often called "shock."

Indígena (Spanish) — A native American or Indian.

Kinetic energy — The energy of motion.

Latex — The sticky, milky sap of certain plants, which yields natural rubber when heated and coagulated.

Limbic forebrain — A part of the evolutionarily old brain containing centers of pain and pleasure; also associated with memory and emotion. It is possible that this area of the brain is involved in altered states of consciousness, highs, and responses to psychoactive drugs.

Lime — Calcium oxide (quicklime) or calcium hydroxide (slaked lime) — caustic minerals that form strongly alkaline solutions and have wide use in chemistry and industry. Not to be confused with the citrus fruit.

LSD — Lysergic acid diethylamide, a potent hallucinogenic drug synthesized from a compound occurring naturally in ergot, the fungus that attacks rye and other grains

Luminescence — "Cold light." The production of light without heat by electronically excited molecules. Luminescence occurs in physical, chemical, and biological systems. Bioluminescence can be seen in a wide range of species, from certain mushrooms and plankton to certain clams and insects.

Macrobiotics — A dietary system invented in Japan in the twentieth century that emphasizes whole grains, especially brown rice, and urges avoidance of foods classified as strongly yin or yang (q.v.).

Maestro (Spanish) — Teacher.

Maguey (pronounced mah-GAY) — Any of several large desert plants of the New World, of the genus *Agave* in the lily family. Varieties of century plants, they have thick, swordlike leaves that develop from a central cone. The sap of magueys is the basis of several native Mexican alcoholic beverages, including *pulque, mezcal,* and *tequila.*

Mandrake — *Mandragora officinarum,* an Old World plant of the nightshade family, containing tropane alkaloids and used in European witchcraft of the Middle Ages.

Medulla oblongata — The lowest structure of the brainstem (q.v.), forming a link between the pons above and the spinal cord below. It contains nerve centers controlling heartbeat and breathing.

Methadone — A synthetic, long-acting narcotic, used in treatment programs to maintain heroin addicts. Taken orally, it gives little euphoria and blocks the effect of heroin. Withdrawal from methadone can be more difficult than withdrawal from heroin.

Muscimol — The psychoactive principle of the Fly Agaric, *Amanita muscaria.* It produces a dreamy intoxication, sometimes with periods of excitement.

Muscular dystrophy — A group of disorders of unknown cause, leading to incapacitation through progressive deterioration of muscle tissue.

Mycology — That branch of biology that studies fungi, including mushrooms.

Mycophile — (Literally, "fungus lover.") One who loves or enjoys mushrooms.

Mycophobe — (Literally, "fungus hater.") One who fears or shuns mushrooms.

Narcotic — A stupor-inducing drug, derived from opium or chemically related to the compounds in opium. Narcotics depress central nervous system functioning and, in chronic use, can produce a dependence syndrome marked by tolerance (q.v.) and withdrawal (q.v.).

Naturopath — Practitioner of a system of healing that relies on dietetics, massage, applications of heat and cold, baths, and the use of vitamin and mineral supplements.

Neurotransmission — The conveyance of impulses along nerve pathways by electrical and chemical means.

Nightshade — Any plant belonging to the Solanaceae, the nightshade or potato family. Specifically, the Deadly Nightshade, *Atropa belladonna*. Tomatoes, potatoes, eggplants, and chilies are members of this group, along with a number of more dangerous plants, such as tobacco and *Datura*.

Oaxaca (pronounced wah-HAH-kah) — A state of southern Mexico, mostly desert, with a large Indian population. Also the capital city of that state.

Ophthalmology — That branch of medicine that studies and treats diseases of the eyes.

Panaeolus — A genus of dung-inhabiting mushrooms with black spores. Several species contain the hallucinogenic drug psilocybin.

Parasympathetic blockade — Paralysis of nerves of the parasympathetic nervous system (q.v.), usually a temporary condition due to the action of a parasympathetic-blocking drug.

Parasympathetic nervous system — That branch of the autonomic nervous system (q.v.) that tends to slow down body functions and promote relaxation. Nerves of this system leave the head and lower part of the spine and connect to numerous organs, blood vessels, and glands.

Peripheral nervous system — All parts of the nervous system other than the brain and spinal cord.

Peyote — A small, spineless cactus, *Lophophora williamsii*, native to north-central Mexico and adjacent areas of Texas and New Mexico. Peyote contains several dozen alkaloids, of which mescaline is the most important. Many North American Indians eat peyote ceremonially for its psychedelic effect.

Procaine — A synthetic local anesthetic, marketed under the brand name Novocain.

Psilocybin — A strong hallucinogenic drug occurring naturally in a number of species of mushrooms. It produces an intoxication marked by colored visions, lasting four to six hours.

Psyche — The mind as opposed to the body.

Psychedelic — (Literally, "mind-manifesting.") A drug, such as LSD, mescaline, or psilocybin, that, under appropriate conditions of set and setting, can elicit high states marked by philosophic insights, mystical feelings, visions, and so forth. The term reflects a positive bias toward these drugs, which others have less kindly called "hallucinogens" (hallucination inducers) or "psychotomimetics" (psychosis mimickers).

Psychoactive — Affecting the mind, especially mood, thought, or perception. Referring to drugs or plants with these effects.

Psychokinesis — The power of affecting physical reality by purely mental means, such as willing dice to come up a certain way or causing objects to move or break.

Psychophysiology — The functioning of the body in its interactions with mind; also the expressions of mind through the physical body, especially by way of nerves, hormones, and so forth. Also, the study of these phenomena.

Psychosis — Loss of ability to distinguish reality, as perceived by others, from one's own private mental productions. The most serious category of mental illness, often marked by hallucinations, delusions, and disturbances of thought and mood.

Psychotropic — (Literally, "mind-turning.") Affecting the mind, especially its functions of mood, thought, and perception. Applied to certain drugs and plants. Equivalent to "psychoactive."

Ramada (Spanish) — A shed, hut, or shelter, especially one made of branches.

Sabroso (Spanish) — Rich in flavor.

Sahuaro — The giant columnar cactus, *Carnegiea gigantea* (or *Cereus giganteus*), of southern Arizona and adjacent Mexico. Also spelled "saguaro."

Set — Expectation, especially unconscious expectation, as a variable that determines people's reactions to drugs and other stimuli.

Setting — Environment — physical, social, and cultural — as a variable that determines people's reactions to drugs and other stimuli.

Shaman — A priest or medicine man who mediates personally between the human world and spirit world and often attempts to control the forces of good and evil within a tribal community. Shamanism is common among native peoples of northern Asia and North and South America. It frequently involves the use of psychoactive plants to induce altered states of consciousness conducive to magical operations.

Smooth muscle — Involuntary muscle, such as in the stomach, intestines, and uterus, controlled by nerves of the autonomic nervous system (q.v.). Opposed to striated (or striped) muscle, which is under voluntary control.

Solanaceae (Solanaceous, adj.) — The nightshade family (q.v.) of flowering plants.

Soma — The body as opposed to the mind. Also, the name of a psychoactive drink used ritually and religiously by the Aryan peoples of the Indian subcontinent in ancient times. Its exact botanical identification is still the subject of speculation.

Spore — An asexual, reproductive cell of lower plants and fungi.

Stimulant — Any substance that increases activity in the nervous system. Central nervous system stimulants cause wakefulness, alertness, and feelings of well-being. In overdose they may cause anxiety, jitteriness, and insomnia.

Stipe — The stemlike part of a mushroom.

Stupor — A state of reduced sensibility, marked by lethargy and mental confusion. Drugs that depress the central nervous system can cause stupor in high doses.

Sutra — In Buddhism, a sacred text, especially one believed to be a discourse of the Buddha.

Sympathetic nervous system — That branch of the autonomic nervous system (q.v.) that mobilizes the body for fight or flight by speeding up heartbeat and breathing while shutting down digestive functions. Nerves of this system leave the middle segments of the spinal cord to connect to many organs, blood vessels, and glands.

Synergism — In pharmacology, the interaction of two drugs to produce a combined effect greater than the simple sum of their individual effects.

Tannins — Bitter-tasting chemicals derived from the barks, leaves, and fruits of many plants that have the property of tanning animal hides to leather

Taoist — Follower of the philosophy of Taoism, an ancient Chinese system founded by Lao Tzu and outlined in his brief text, the *Tao*

Teh Ching (Way of Life). Taoism stresses the complementary interaction of opposite forces (called yin and yang, q.v.).

Tarot — A deck of cards depicting traditional Western occult philosophy in symbolic, pictorial form. The most important cards of
the deck are twenty-two major trumps, mostly showing human
or supernatural figures. Tarot cards are also used in fortune-
telling, and modern playing cards are derived from them.

Telepathy — Direct mind-to-mind transmission or reception of information.

Tolerance — In pharmacology, the need for increasing doses of a
drug over time to maintain the same effect. Tolerance is a common characteristic of dependence on drugs. It is provoked by
some drugs more than others, especially by stimulants and depressants of the central nervous system.

Tremor — An involuntary shaking or trembling of a part of the
body, such as the hand. Tremor is usually a symptom of dysfunc-
tion of the central nervous system.

Tropane alkaloids — A group of toxic and psychoactive drugs found
in a number of species of plants of the nightshade family (q.v.).
Atropine and scopolamine are the most important.

Vanillin — A chemical occurring naturally in the vanilla bean and
largely responsible for its flavor. Synthetic vanillin is much
cheaper than vanilla bean but does not exactly reproduce the
complex flavor of the natural product.

Withdrawal syndrome — Any cluster of symptoms that appears
when a drug that has been taken regularly is stopped and that
disappears when the drug is reinstituted. Withdrawal syndromes
are a characteristic of certain kinds of drug dependence, especially dependence on depressants of the central nervous system,
like alcohol, opiates, and barbiturates.

Xanthines — A group of related alkaloids found in various plants
that stimulate the central nervous system. Caffeine in coffee,
theophylline in tea, and theobromine in chocolate are examples.

Yaqui — One of the Yaquis, a tribe of Indians of the Sonoran desert
in northwest Mexico.

Yarumo Blanco (Spanish) — A type of cecropia tree, large trees of
the fig family found throughout the Amazon basin.

Yin and yang — The fundamental opposite forces central to the philosophy of Taoism and Chinese thought. Yin is the receptive, feminine element, associated with earth; yang the creative, masculine element associated with heaven. These two forces are locked together in perpetual, antagonistic, complementary interaction.

Yoga — (Literally "union.") An ancient system, developed in India, of physical and mental practices designed to expand human consciousness and reunite man with God.

Yogi — A practitioner of yoga.

SUGGESTED READING

ON THE ROLE OF THE AUTONOMIC NERVOUS SYSTEM

Cannon, Walter B. *The Wisdom of the Body.* New York: W. W. Norton & Co., 1963 (first published in 1932).

Pelletier, Kenneth R. *Mind as Healer, Mind as Slayer.* New York: Bantam, Doubleday, Dell, 1992.

ON PSYCHOACTIVE PLANTS

Schultes, Richard Evans, and Albert Hofmann. *Plants of the Gods: Origins of Hallucinogenic Use.* New York: McGraw Hill, 1979.

Weil, Andrew, and Winifred Rosen. *From Chocolate to Morphine: Everything You Need to Know About Mind-Altering Drugs* (rev. ed.). Boston: Houghton Mifflin, 2004.

ON PLANTS OF THE NIGHTSHADE FAMILY

Hansen, Harold A. *The Witch's Garden.* Santa Cruz, California: Unity Press, 1978.

Heiser, Charles B. *Nightshades: The Pardoxical Plants.* San Francisco: W. H. Freeman & Co., 1969.

ON THE THERAPEUTIC VALUE OF LAUGHTER

Cousins, Norman. *Anatomy of an Illness (As Perceived by the Patient).* New York: W. W. Norton & Co., 1979.

Moody, Raymond A., Jr. *Laugh After Laugh: The Healing Power of Humor.* Jacksonville, Florida: Headwaters Press, 1978.

ON PSYCHEDELIC MUSHROOMS

Stamets, Paul. *Psilocybin Mushrooms of the World: An Identification Guide.* Berkeley, California: Ten Speed Press, 1996.

Metzner, Ralph (ed.), with Diane Conn Darling. *Teonanácatl: Sacred Mushroom of Visions.* El Verano, California: Green Earth Foundation Books, 2003.

Riedlinger, Thomas J. (ed.). *The Sacred Mushroom Seeker: Essays for R. Gordon Wasson*. Portland, Oregon: Dioscorides Press, 1990.

ON MARIJUANA

Grinspoon, Lester. *Marihuana Reconsidered* (reprint ed.). San Francisco: Quick Trading Co., 1994.

Pollan, Michael. *The Botany of Desire: A Plant's Eye View of the World*. New York: Random House, 2002.

Schlosser, Eric. *Reefer Madness: Sex, Drugs, and Cheap Labor in the American Black Market*. Boston: Houghton Mifflin, 2003.

ON YAGÉ

Metzner, Ralph, Dennis McKenna, Charles S. Grob, and Jace Calloway. *Ayahuasca: Hallucinogens, Consciousness, and the Spirits of Nature*. New York: Thunder's Mouth Press, 1999.

Wilcox, Joan Parisi. *Ayahuasca: The Visionary and Healing Powers of the Vine of the Soul*. Rochester, Vermont: Inner Traditions International, 2003.

Luna, Luis Eduardo, and Steven F. White (eds.). *Ayahuasca Reader: Encounters with the Amazon's Sacred Vine*. Santa Fe, New Mexico: Synergetic Press, 2000.

Lamb, F. Bruce, and Manuel C. Rios. *Kidnapped in the Amazon Jungle*. Berkeley, California: North Atlantic Books, 1994.

ON COCOA AND COCAINE

Andrews, George, and David Solomon (eds.). *The Coca Leaf and Cocaine Papers*. New York: Harcourt Brace Jovanovich, 1975.

Antonil, *Mama Coca*. London: Hassle Free Press, 1978.

Mortimer, W. Golden. *History of Coca: Divine Plant of the Incas*. San Francisco: And/Or Press, 1974 (first published in 1901).

Leons, Madeline Barbara, and Harry Sanabria (eds.). *Coca, Cocaine, and the Bolivian Reality*. Albany: State University of New York Press, 1997.

ON MDA AND OTHER PSYCHEDELIC DRUGS

Holland, Julie (ed.). *Ecstasy The Complete Guide: A Comprehensive Look at the Risks and Benefits of MDMA*. Rochester, Vermont: Inner Traditions International, 2001.

Stafford, Peter. *Psychedelics*. Berkeley, California: Ronin Publishing, 2003.

Weil, Andrew, and Winifred Rosen. *From Chocolate to Morphine: Everything You Need to Know About Mind-Altering Drugs* (rev. ed.). Boston: Houghton Mifflin, 2004.

ON ALTERNATIVE MEDICINE

Weil, Andrew. *Health and Healing* (rev. ed.). Boston: Houghton Mifflin, 2004.

ON URI GELLER

Panati, Charles (ed.). *The Geller Papers*. Boston: Houghton Mifflin, 1976.
Randi, The Amazing. *The Magic of Uri Geller*. New York: Ballantine Books, 1972.

ON SOLAR ECLIPSES

Littmann, Mark, and Ken Willcox. *Totality: Eclipses of the Sun*. Honolulu: University of Hawaii Press, 1991.

ON ALTERED STATES OF CONSCIOUSNESS AND HIGHS

Weil, Andrew. *The Natural Mind: A New Way of Looking and Drugs and the Higher Consciousness* (rev. ed.). Boston: Houghton Mifflin, 2004.

ON THE SIOUX SWEAT LODGE AND OTHER RITUALS

Halifax, Joan (ed.). *Shamanic Voices: A Survey of Visionary Narratives* (reissue ed.). New York: Penguin, 1994.
Lame Deer, John (Fire). *Lame Deer, Seeker of Visions: The Life of a Sioux Medicine Man* (rev. ed.). New York: Simon & Schuster, 1994.
Mails, Thomas E. *Sundancing at Rosebud and Pine Ridge*. Sioux Falls, South Dakota: Center for Western Studies, 1978.

INDEX

Abend, Martin, 209, 211–12, 218
Active principles, 17, 97, 142, 162–63, 165
Addiction, 18, 19, 20, 34; and sugar, 135–37; and coca, 157; and cocaine, 158
Addictive potential, 18
Addicts, 136, 137, 159
Africa, 224, 226–33
Agaricus brunnescens, 58, 63
Agaricus campestris, 58–59
Agua de coca, 163
Aguardiente, 113, 114–15, 116, 119, 120, 121, 123, 124, 127, 128, 129, 131
Alchemy, 244
Alcohol, 19, 37, 41, 111, 113, 128, 129, 179; and Indians, 130; and Uri Geller, 198; *see also* Aguardiente; Chicha; Guarapo; Rum
Alcoholic gastritis, 33
Alcoholics Anonymous, 19
Alexander, Robert, 41
Algonquins, 172–73
Alkalies, 142–43, 148, 163
Alkaloids, 80, 101, 109, 162–63, 167–68; *see also* Atropine; Caffeine; Cocaine; DMT; Harmaline; Heroin; Mescaline;

Morphine; Muscarine; Psilocybin; Scopolamine; Tropane Alkaloids; Xanthines
Allergy, 180
Allopathy, 182, 183, 189
Altered states of consciousness. *See* Consciousness, altered states of
Amanita muscaria, 43, 45–47, 71
Amanita pantherina. See Panther Amanita
Amanita phalloides, 47, 69
Amanitas, 43, 45–47, 61, 67, 68–69, 71, 79–82; *illus.*, 78
Amazon basin, 55, 107, 108, 113, 117, 125, 129–30, 142, 145
Ambrosio, 126–29
Amnesia, 109, 168–69, 170, 175
Amphetamines, 18n, 140, 177
Andes, 57, 105, 129, 142, 144, 145, 173
Anergy, 180
Anesthesia, 140, 144, 148, 157, 158, 163, 251–52
Anise, 61, 113, 117, 123
Antikinetic action, 177–78
Argentina, 15, 142
Arizona, 73, 166
Armoring, 183

Aryans, 43
Asia, 25, 28, 254
Asthma, 17, 96, 180
Astronomers, 233
Atropine, 80, 81, 109, 167–68
Attention, 26, 232, 253
Autobiography of a Yogi
    (Yogananda), 25
Ayahuasca. *See* Yagé
Aztecs, 29

Babies, 39, 169–70
Back to Eden (Kloss), 33
Bactris gasipaës, 149n
Baking soda, 143
Banisteriopsis caapi. See Yagé
Belladonna, 94, 109, 167
Blindfolds, 195
Blindness: and solar eclipses,
    224–26, 233, 236–37
Blue Halos. *See Psilocybe
    cyanescens*
Bogotá, 56, 102, 103, 107, 139,
    141, 145, 153, 157, 219
Boletes, 59, 61
Boletus edulis, 61
Bolivia, 142, 143, 144
Bombay, 25, 26
Book of Changes, 70
Borana, 227–28, 233
Brain, 9, 10, 184, 251, 256; left
    and right, 256–57
Brainstem, 9, 38–39, 40, 257
Brazil, 15, 145
Breasts, 93
Breathing, 12, 39
Brugmansia. See Tree Datura
Brujos, 101, 107, 113, 118; *see
    also* Witch doctors
Buddhists, 255, 256
Burroughs, William, 101

Caapi. *See* Yagé
Cacao, 15, 16, 165; *illus.*, 16
Café, 16
Caffeine, 15–21, 140
Caffeine-nicotine syndrome, 19,
    177
California, 76, 118, 123, 166, 182,
    184, 185, 191, 192, 196, 257
California Psychical Research
    Society, 192
Calories, 65, 68
Camels, 227, 229, 230
Canada, 84, 235–37
Canadian Broadcasting Com-
    mission, 237
Cancer, 97
Cannabis. *See* Marijuana
Cantharellus cibarius. See Chan-
    terelles
Cap of Liberty, 77
Capsaicin, 31
Capsicum, 28–36, 51, 146, 149;
    illus., 29, 30, 35
Carson, Johnny, 201, 203, 214
Carter, Josh, 184–87, 188
Casave, 146, 149, 153
Cashew family, 24n
Castaneda, Carlos, 173, 221, 256
Cauca, 68, 144
Cayenne pepper, 28
Cecropia, 149–50, 153
Cerebral hemispheres, 38, 39, 40,
    256–57
Cerebral palsy, 97
Chagrapanga, 111, 114, 116, 119,
    126, 127, 128; *illus.*, 112
Chalbi Desert, 226–31
Chamico, 172
Chanterelles, 58, 61, 63, 64, 71,
    83; *illus.*, 64
Chanting, 114, 121, 243; and

sweat lodge, 249, 251; and pain, 252, 253, 254, 255

Chemotherapy, 97

Chicha, 111, 115, 117, 130, 146, 147, 149, 150, 151, 153

Childbirth, 94, 109, 168–70

Children, 258

Chile, 142

Chili, 23, 28–36, 38, 146, 149; in mushroom ceremony, 51; *illus.*, 29, 30, 35

Chiltepín, 29

Chindoy, Salvador, 107–17; *illus.*, 108

Chinese philosophy, 68, 70

Chocolate, 15, 29, 165; *illus.*, 16

Choking, 258

Cholesterol, 137

Coca, 55, 139–65; occurrence of, 142; and Indians, 142–58, 163; method of use of, 143, 148; flavor of, 143; and physical work, 144; preparation of by Cubeos, 147, 149, 153–54; *illus.*, 150, 152, 154, 155, 156; and health, 145, 157, 163–64; and dependence, 157, 164; versus cocaine, 157–58, 162–63; nutritional value of, 163–64

Coca-Cola, 164

Cocada, 144

Cocaine, 139–42; classification of, 140, 158; cost of, 140; effects of, 140–41; versus coca, 157–58, 162–63; and health, 158–61; depression following use of, 159–60; and heroin, 159, 164; dependence on, 160–61; and nasal membranes, 160–61

Cocoa, 15, 165; *illus.*, 16

Cocoa butter, 15

Coffee, 15–21, 90, 93, 139, 165, 177, 229; *illus.*, 14

Cola, 15, 164

Colegio de Tepoztlán, 5–6

Colombia, 6, 7, 27, 54–56, 60, 68, 99–131, 139–65, 173, 176, 219–20

Columbus, 28

Concentration, 26, 202, 243, 251; and pain, 252–55

Conscious mind. *See* Mind, conscious

Consciousness, 3, 5, 195, 241; revolution in, 86; dualism of, 244–46, 255–59; *see also* Consciousness, altered states of

Consciousness, altered states of, 4, 26, 43, 47, 241–43; and psilocybin mushrooms, 67–68, 75–76; and drugs, 87–88, 115, 165; and scopolamine, 168–70; and eclipses, 224, 231–32, 243–44, 246; mechanisms of, 246, 255, 257; and sweat lodge, 250–51; and medicine, 257; and children, 258

Cooking of India (Rau), 34

Copal, 51

Coprinus comatus. See Shaggy Manes

Córdova-Rios, Manuel, 101

Corona, 223, 224, 231, 232, 243; *illus.*, 223, 235

Cortex, 9, 40, 257

Costa Rica, 23, 27, 176

Cough: from marijuana, 92

Cows, 56–57, 76–77

Crying, 40–41

Cubeos, 145–57; *illus.*, 150, 152, 154, 155, 156

Cuduyarí, 145

Daily Texan, 204–5
Dance, 87, 151, 254
Datura, 120, 166–76; *illus.*, 110, 167, 174; *see also* Tree Datura
Datura inoxia, 166; *illus.*, 167
Datura metel, 172
Datura meteloides, 166, 175; *illus.*, 167
Datura stramonium. See Jimsonweed
Death, 45, 69, 70, 247
Death Cup, 46, 69
Defense Department, 197
Dental caries, 137
Dependence, 18, 19, 20, 21, 34, 91, 92, 157, 158, 159, 160
Derealization, 222, 243
Desires, 178–79
Devil, 199
Dhatureas, 172
Diagnosis, 182, 184, 185, 189
Diagnosis from the Eye (Liljequist), 181
Diamond ring, 231; *illus.*, 223
Diaphragm, 37, 40
Dimethyltryptamine. *See* DMT
Diplopterys cabrerana. See Chagrapanga
Diuretics, 17
DMT, 101, 111
DNA, 184
Don Juan, 173, 221, 256
Dopamine, 255
Dreams, 70, 122, 169, 232, 243, 256
Dream yoga, 256, 259
Drowning, 172
Drug abuse, 164–65
Drugs, 1, 3, 4, 5; and Indians, 3, 130–31; and nausea, 11; and highs, 87–88, 242; relationships with, 89–92; frequency of use of, 90–91; education about, 165; and powers, 201; and altered states of consciousness, 232, 243, 259; fears of, 247; and pain, 252–53; *see also* specific drugs
Drugs, hallucinogenic: and nausea, 8, 11; and highs, 57, 179; *see also* DMT; LSD; MDA; Mescaline; Peyote; Psilocybin; Psilocybin mushrooms; Yagé
Duba, 228, 229, 230

Earth: alignment of with sun and moon, 232
East African Standard, 233
Eclipses, lunar, 53, 229
Eclipses, solar, 5, 222–40, 243–44; effects of on consciousness, 224, 231–32, 243–44; and eye damage, 224, 225–26, 229, 233–34, 235–37; phobia of, 225–26, 228, 243, 247; governmental responses to, 225, 226, 228, 233–34, 235–37; *illus.*, 223, 235, 238–39
Ecuador, 57, 105, 130, 142, 160, 173, 175
Ego, 39, 43, 255
Eldorado Airport, 139
Eleusinian mysteries, 43
El Molo, 233
Emotions, 11, 39, 40, 251
Empire State Building, 237; *illus.*, 239
Energy, 183, 197, 204, 253, 255; of mushrooms, 65–71; solar, 68, 70; lunar, 69–71, 78, 247; and cocaine, 159; and MDA, 179; and matter, 195; and consciousness, 195
Enlightenment, 41, 244

Epilepsy, 40, 97
Equilibrium, 232
Erythroxylum. See Coca
Eskimos, 102
ESP, 209; *see also* Telepathy
Espeletia, 106
Ethiopia, 15, 227
Eucharist, 51
Eugene, Oregon, 58, 59, 73, 76, 83, 85, 218
Eugene Mycological Society, 61
Evergreen State College, 84
Expectation. *See* Set
Experience, 241
Experiment, 241
Eye, 38, 163, 181–89; and solar eclipses, 224, 225–26, 229, 233–34, 235–37

Faith, 221, 250
Falling sickness, 40; *see also* Epilepsy
False Chanterelle, 61
Fantasy, 221
Fasting, 87
Fire, 68, 246, 248, 250, 252, 253, 254–55
Fire walking, 4, 254–55
First World Congress of Sorcery, 219
Fits. *See* Laughing fits
Florida, 25, 55, 224
Fly Agaric. *See Amanita muscaria*
Fly Amanita. *See Amanita muscaria*
Flying saucers, 205, 207
Food, and vomiting, 12
Freud, Sigmund, 157
Freudians, 183, 256, 257

Gabra, 226–31
Galerina, 82

Geller, Uri, 191–221; *illus.*, 190; introduced, 192; performs telepathy, 193, 197, 205–6, 209–10; beliefs of, 198–99; bends metal, 199–201, 210–11; accused of fraud, 203–4; 219; evaluated by James Randi, 212–18; conclusions about, 220
Ghost Dance, 234
Glaucoma, 96
Gold, 244
Great Spirit, 248
Griffin, Merv, 195, 201, 214, 215
Group encounter, 40
Guamués, 106
Guaraná, 15
Guarapo, 132–33
Guatemala, 15, 23
Gynecomastia, 93

Haight-Ashbury, 101
Hallucinations, 52, 63, 179; of mushrooms, 76; and Datura, 170–71
Hallucinogens. *See* Drugs, hallucinogenic
Harmaline, 101, 102
Harner, Michael, 175
Harvard Botanical Museum, 99
Hawaiians, 199
Headache, 11, 95, 209
Headstand, 178
Healing, 4, 33; and hallucinogenic drugs, 57; and Uri Geller, 199, 203, 204, 220
Healing Journey (Naranjo), 102
Health, 39, 41, 188, 259; and high states, 87; and drug use, 92; and marijuana, 92; and coca, 145, 157; and cocaine, 158, 160–61; and sweat lodge, 250
Heat, 248–52

Hemp. *See* Marijuana
Henbane, 109, 167
Herbal medicine, 32–33
Hermes, 181
Heroin, 18, 135–38, 140, 159, 162, 164
High Priestess, 245
Highs, 3, 4, 5; and pain, 26, 34, 36, 251–55, 257; and chilies, 34, 36; and laughter, 40; and mushrooms, 46; and drugs, 87–92, 95, 136; and cocaine, 140–41, 158; and coca, 144, 151; and MDA, 177; of solar eclipses, 224, 226, 232, 234, 240, 243–44, 246; of sweat lodge, 250–51; evolutionary logic of, 257–58
Hindus, 21, 25, 254
Homeopathy, 95, 181
Hoover, Herbert, 237; *illus.*, 238
Huáutla de Jiménez, 48, 49
Hurricane's eye, 223, 232
Hyenas, 39
Hyman, Ray, 218–19
Hyperventilation, 258
Hypnosis, 4, 169, 232, 251, 253
Hysterical dissociation, 251–52

Ice cream, 12, 197
I Ching, 70
Id, 255
Illness, 9–10, 50, 175; diagnosis of, 182, 184, 185, 189
Imagination, 221
Incas, 32, 107, 144
Incense, 51, 124, 248
India, 25–26, 28, 34–35, 172
Indians, 3, 20, 30, 48, 119, 166; and drugs, 3, 130–31; Sioux, 5, 248–50, 252; Papagos, 8–9; Mazatec, 48–50; Colombian, 99; Amahuaca, 101, 114; In-

ganos, 107–8, 120, 173; Kamsas, 107–8, 119, 173; Mocoas, 126–29; debasement of cultures of, 129–30; Kofanes, 130; and psychoactive plants, 130–31; and alcohol, 130, 132–33; and coca, 142–43, 144–57; Cubeos, 145–57; and Datura, 172–75; Algonquins, 172–73; Jívaros, 175; and solar eclipses, 222, 224; Paiute, 234
Inganos, 107–8, 120, 173
Ingas. *See* Inganos
Injections, 49–50
Inky Caps, 61, 65
Insomnia, 94, 95
Institute of Current World Affairs, 2
Intellect, 244, 259
Intuition, 44, 45, 70, 257; and diagnosis, 189
Iridology, 181–88; *illus.*, 186–87
Iris (goddess), 181, 184
Iris (of eye), 181–88; *illus.*, 186–87

Jack-O'-Lantern Mushroom, 67
Jalapeño peppers, 29; *illus.*, 29, 35
Japanese, 255
Jaroff, Leon, 221
Jensen, Bernard, 184–85, 186–87
Jimsonweed, 109, 119, 166–67, 172; origin of name, 172
Jívaros, 175
Julieta, 49–54
Justice Department, 225, 226, 233, 234

Kamsas, 107–8, 119, 173; *illus.*, 108
Katz, Jascha, 196, 198, 208, 211
Kenya, 226, 227, 233

King Boletus, 61
Kloss, Jethro, 33
Kofanes, 130
Koller, Karl, 157

Lacrimal glands, 38, 39
Lacrimation, 38, 39; and vomit-
  ing, 12; and chilies, 34
Lactarius sanguifluus, 64
Language learning, 5–6
La Paz, 142, 143
Latin America, 5, 15, 47, 74, 132,
  133, 136; *see also* Colombia;
  Costa Rica; Ecuador;
  Guatemala; Mexico; Peru
Laughing fits, 37–42
Laughing gas. *See* Nitrous oxide
Laughter, 37–42, 126–29; and
  psilocybin mushrooms, 75
Left, 257
Levitation, 208
Lianas, 99n, 103; *illus.*, 100
Liberty Cap, 73–79, 82, 83, 84, 85;
  origin of name, 77; *illus.*, 72
Liljequist, Nils, 181
Limbic forebrain, 255
Lime, 143
Lockwood, Tommie, 175
LSD, 5, 57, 63, 101, 123, 252
Luminescence, 67
Lunacy, 69, 78, 247
Lunar energy, 69–71, 79, 247

Machaca, 125
Macrobiotics, 68, 69
Magic, 20, 50, 54, 57, 166, 175,
  202, 247
Magician, 245
Magicians, 166, 195, 203, 204,
  212–18
Maguey, 6
Mama Coca, 142, 163, 165

Mandrake, 167
Mangoes, 23–27; *illus.*, 22, 24
Manitoba, 235–37
Manitoba Medical Association,
  236
Marijuana, 20, 21, 41, 55, 81,
  87–98, 111, 115, 140, 160, 179;
  physical effects of, 88; and
  health, 92–93; as a remedy,
  93–98; illegality of, 98; *illus.*,
  88, 89, 94
Marriage of the sun and moon, 5,
  244; *illus.*, 242
Martial arts, 178
Martin, Richard, 157, 162
Martyr, Peter, 28
Massage, 183
Maté, 15
Materialists, 255
Matter, and energy, 195
Mayans, 32
Mazatecs, 48–50
MDA, 57, 177–80, 252
Meadow Mushrooms, 58–59, 83
Medicine: Chinese, 183, 185; or-
  thodox, 240; unorthodox, 189
Medicine man, 248, 249, 251
Meditation, 4, 5, 26, 44, 87, 169,
  198, 202, 232, 259
Medulla oblongata, 9, 10, 38
Men, 93
Mercury, 223
Mescaline, 57
Metal bending, 191, 194, 195,
  198, 199–201, 204–5, 206–7,
  208, 210–11; by sleight-of-
  hand, 203, 215, 217; *illus.*, 190
Methadone, 136
Mexico, 5–7, 9, 13, 20, 23, 29, 30,
  32, 43, 47–54, 55, 56, 62, 132,
  166, 170–71, 175, 222–25, 226,
  232–33

Miahuatlán, 222, 224, 231
Midbrain, 38
Milky caps, 61, 64
Mind: conscious, 39, 245; day, 39,
44, 244–45; lunar, 244–46, 247,
254, 255, 256, 257, 258, 259;
night, 39, 44, 45, 245; solar,
244–46, 247, 251, 253, 254, 255,
256, 259; unconscious, 39–40,
45, 70, 71, 78, 169, 245, 246,
255–56
Mind-body relationships, 39, 40,
96, 183, 250–59
Miracles, 191, 196, 208
Mitchell, Edgar, 205
Mocoa, 117, 118, 120, 124, 126,
130
Mocoa Indians, 126–29
Molasses, 133, 134
Montalban, Ricardo, 201
Montaña, 142
Moon, 50, 53, 68, 70, 205, 222,
231, 245–46; eclipses of, 53,
229; and mushrooms, 68, 70,
246–47; alignment of earth and
sun with, 232, 243–44; as sym-
bol, 245; goddess, 245
Mormons, 20
Morphine, 136, 162
Morris, Desmond, 40
Motion sickness, 11, 97
"Mouth surfing," 34
Multiple sclerosis, 97
Muscarine, 80
Muscles, 97, 122, 151, 178,
182–84, 253, 255; and nerves,
182–83; of iris, 182, 184, 185
Mushroom cloud, 45n
Mushrooms, 43–86, 246–47;
poisoning by, 43, 79–82, 247;
cultivated, 43, 47, 58; hunting

for, 60, 71, 74–75, 77; taste of,
51–52, 53, 69, 74, 75; learning
about, 62; nutritional value of,
65–68, 70–71; deadly, 67, 69;
and sun, 68; and moon, 68, 70,
246–47; and water, 68; and yin
energy, 68–70; Chinese black,
86; Oyster, 86; *illus.*, 46, 64, 66,
72, 78, 85; *see also* Mushrooms,
magic; Psilocybin mushrooms;
specific mushrooms
Mushrooms, magic, 7, 43–57, 115,
126, 246–47; *illus.*, 46, 72, 85;
see also Psilocybin mushrooms
Music, 87, 150, 151, 154, 158
Muslims, 21
Mycologists, 62, 79, 83
Mycophiles, 43, 58, 59
Mycophilia, 65
Mycophobes, 43, 59
Mycophobia, 43, 247
Mysteries, 43

Naked Ape (Morris), 40
Naranjo, Claudio, 102
Narcotics, 158, 159, 162; *see also*
Heroin; Methadone; Mor-
phine; Opiates; Opium
Narendra, 25
National Institute of Mental
Health, 21
National Society for the Preven-
tion of Blindness, 225
Natural Mind (Weil), 1, 3, 4,
241–43, 257–58
Nausea, 5, 81, 82, 177; and mari-
juana, 96–97; and yagé, 122;
and opium, 136, 137
Nervous system, 4, 10, 13, 27, 79,
87, 88, 159, 182–83, 184,
253–56, 259; autonomic, 9–10,

12, 38–40; central, 17, 97, 168, 253; involuntary, 9, 38; parasympathetic, 9–10, 38–39, 80, 167–68; peripheral, 253–54
New Scientist, 205
New World, 15, 28, 29, 32, 166, 172, 173
New York, 205, 221
Niemann, Albert, 157
Nightshade family, 28, 80, 109, 119, 166, 167, 173, 175
Nitrous oxide, 41
Nolte, Richard, 2

Oaxaca, 7, 20, 31, 48–54, 222–24
Obesity, 137
Oceanic feelings, 257
Odell, Charles M., 225
Oil, 129–31
Old World, 15, 28, 142, 166
Ophthalmologists, 188, 236
Opiates, 158–59, 162, 170, 251; see also Heroin; Methadone; Morphine
Opium, 94, 136, 137, 162
Oregon, 58–64, 73–86
Oregon State University, 76
Ornstein, Robert, 44
Owls, 181, 186

Paar, Jack, 195
Pacific Northwest, 58, 79, 80; *see also* Oregon; Washington (state)
Pain, 26, 34, 36, 37, 169, 183; nonhurtful, 178, 251–55, 257
Palo santo, 51
Panaeolus subbalteatus, 82
Panama, 27
Pan American Highway, 105, 113, 144

Panela, 133, 134, 137, 138, 162, 163
Panic reactions, 57
Panther Amanita, 68–69, 71, 79–82; *illus.*, 78
Papagos, 8–9
Páramos, 106
Pasta (cocaine), 160
Patanjali, 201
Patu, 147–48
PCP, 63
Peach Palm, 149n
Peczely, Ignatz von, 181, 186
Pedro, 118–24
Pepper, black, 28
Pepper, red. *See* Chili
Peru, 56, 114, 142, 172, 173
Peyote, 57, 101, 115
Pharmacologists, 17, 18, 162, 164
Pharmacology, 21
Phencyclidine. *See* PCP
Philadelphia, 24, 37, 51, 77
Photographers, 232, 233
Phrygian bonnet, 77
Physicians, 17, 20, 81, 95, 163, 164, 180, 189, 257
Pielroja (cigarettes), 119
Pig's Ears, 64
Pinhole projection device, 225–26
Pleasure, 26
Poison ivy, 24n
Poisons, 45, 79; mushroom, 43, 47, 67, 68–69, 71, 79–82
Polansky, Marco, 5–6
Pons, 38
Popayán, 144
Pot. *See* Marijuana
Potato family. *See* Nightshade family
Procaine, 140

Psilocybe, 47, 54, 55, 76, 77, 78, 82–86; *illus.* 46, 72, 85; *see also* Liberty Cap; *Psilocybe cubensis;* specific Psilocybes
Psilocybe baeocystis, 83
Psilocybe cubensis, 47, 50–54, 60, 68, 83; cultivation of, 86; *illus.*, 46, 85
Psilocybe cyanescens, 83
Psilocybe semilanceata. See Liberty Cap
Psilocybe stuntzii, 83–84
Psilocybin, 47, 86; *see also* Psilocybin mushrooms
Psilocybin mushrooms, 47–57, 61–63, 67–68, 71, 73–79, 81, 82–86; and lunar energy, 71; visions of, 76, 84; cultivation of, 86; *illus*, 46, 72, 85
Psychedelics, 45, 123, 250; *see also* Drugs, hallucinogenic
Psychiatrists, 255–56, 257, 258
Psychic phenomena, 201–2, 211, 218–19, 220–21; *see also* Metal bending; Psychokinesis; Telepathy
Psychogenic tearing, 39
Psychokinesis, 191, 194, 195, 201, 207, 208, 220; *see also* Metal bending
Psychologists, 255
Psychology of Consciousness (Ornstein), 44
Psychology Today, 219
Psychosomatic disease, 96
Puharich, Andrija, 192, 195, 196, 205
Pulque, 6
Pupuña, 149
Putumayo (river) 106, 126; *illus.*, 125

Putumayo Territory, 101, 102, 106, 107, 117, 125, 126, 129, 130

Quinoa, 143

Raja Yoga (Vivekananda), 191
Ramakrishna, 25
Randi, James (The Amazing), 203–4, 212–18, 220; *illus.*, 214
Rau, Santha Rama, 34
Reality, 221, 232, 243
Real Paper, 207
Red pepper. *See* Chili
Refining, 136, 137–38, 162
Reflex tearing, 38
Reich, Wilhelm, 183, 255–56
Right, 257
Rolf, Ida, 183
Rolfing, 183
Rolling Stone, 207, 208, 209
Rosebud Reservation, 250
Rum, 134
Rumiyaco, 126, 127

Sabina, Maria, 48
Sacred Datura. *See Datura meteloides*
Sahuaros, 8–9
Samburu, 233
Sandflies, 149
San Isidro, 50–51
San Isidro Mushroom. *See Psilocybe cubensis*
San José (Costa Rica), 23
Science and Practice of Iridology (Jensen), 184
Scientists, 203, 216, 232–33
Scopolamine, 109, 167, 168, 171
Secretogogues, 38
Senoi, 256
Set, 3–4, 18, 41, 46, 57, 88; and

Liberty Cap, 79; and Panther Amanita, 81–82; and marijuana, 95, 97; and coca, 165; and MDA, 179; and Uri Geller, 192; and sweat lodge, 251
Setting, 3–4, 41, 57, 165, 179, 251
Sex, 4, 26, 45, 87, 93, 141, 178
Shadow bands, 223, 224
Shaggy Manes, 61, 65–66, 71; *illus.*, 66
Shamans, 130, 173; *see also* Brujos; Chindoy, Salvador; Julieta; Medicine man; Pedro; Witch doctors
Sibundoy, Valley of, 104–5, 106–7, 108, 109, 117, 118, 126, 129, 173; *illus.*, 105
Siddhis, 201–2
Sierra Mazateca, 20, 48, 49, 52
Silver, 244
Sioux, 5, 248–50, 252; *illus.*, 248–49
Skin, 33, 178, 250
Sleight-of-hand, 203, 215, 217
Slippery Jacks, 59–60, 61
Slit lamp, 185
Smoking: of marijuana, 90–91, 92, 96, 98; of tobacco, 91, 119, 120, 150; of cocaine, 160; and MDA, 178–79; of sacred pipe, 248–49
Solanaceae. *See* Nightshade family
Soma, 43
Sonoran Desert, 9
South America, 1, 23, 54–57, 99, 102, 105, 113, 129, 141, 142, 173, 174, 226
Spanish: conquerors, 57, 142; language, 5–6, 49, 107, 110, 146
Spastic paralysis, 97

Speedball, 159
Spinal cord, 9, 38, 97
Spinning, 258
Spores, 86
Stanford Research Institute, 191, 204, 205, 217, 219, 220
Stimulants, 17, 18n; *see also* Caffeine; Coffee; Coca; Cocaine; Drugs, hallucinogenic; Tobacco
Stinkhorns, 45
Stomach, 9, 10, 11, 12, 18, 32, 33
Stropharia cubensis. See Psilocybe cubensis
Stuntz, Daniel, 83
Sucrose, 135, 162
Sugar, 111, 113, 132–38, 162, 229; *see also* Panela
Sugar cane, 113, 132, 133; *illus.*, 133
Sun, 45, 68, 70, 222–40, 245, 246; union of with moon, 232, 244; as symbol, 245; eclipses of. *See* Eclipses, solar
Sweat lodge, 5, 247–52, 254; *illus.*, 248, 249
Sweetness, 136, 137

Tabasco peppers, *illus.*, 30
Tabasco sauce, 32, 36
Tamasic (foods), 70–71
Tapioca, 146
Tarot cards, 245
Tea, 15
Tears. *See* Lacrimation
Telepathine, 101
Telepathy, 101, 123, 191, 193, 197, 201, 205–6, 209–10, 212–13, 220
Television, 225, 226, 234, 236, 237

Temple of Man, 41
Tepozteco, 6, 7
Tepoztlán, 5–7
Testosterone, 93
Tetrahydrocannabinol. *See* THC
Texaco, 129, 130
THC, 97
Theophylline, 17
Tibetans, 256
Time, 224, 231, 243
Time, 192, 195, 218, 221
Toadstools, 43
Tobacco, 19, 91, 93, 109, 119, 121, 150, 160, 165, 177, 178, 248
Tolerance, 160
Toloache, 170–71; *see also* Datura
Toothache, 33
Total eclipses. *See* Eclipses, lunar; Eclipses, solar
Trance, 26, 70, 169, 198, 234, 242, 251
Tranquilizers, 93, 165
Tree Datura, 109, 115, 119, 173, 175; *illus.*, 110, 174
Tremors, 20
Tropane alkaloids, 109, 167–68, 171
Tucson, 176
Turkana, 233
Twain, Mark, 91
Twilight sleep, 109, 168–70

Ulcers, 18, 33, 168
Umbra, 222, 223, 231
Unconscious. *See* Mind, unconscious
University of Washington, 83, 84

Vagus nerve, 9
Vanillin, 31

Vaupés (river), 145
Vaupés Territory, 145, 151
Venus, 223
Virginia, 1, 24, 172, 224, 226
Visions, 56, 76, 78, 84, 114, 119, 122–23, 128, 247, 259
Vitamin C, 31
Vivekananda, 191
Vomiting, 8–13, 97, 121–22, 123
Vomiting center, 9

Washington (state), 62, 80, 83, 84
Washington, D.C., 66, 237
Washington Blue Veil. *See Psilocybe stuntzii*
Wasson, R. Gordon, 43, 48, 53
Water, 68, 69, 246, 250
Wavy Caps. *See Psilocybe cyanescens*
Weil, Mayme, 37
Whipping, 254
Whirling. *See* Spinning
White House, 237; *illus.*, 238
Winnipeg, 236, 237
Wishful thinking, 220–21
Witchcraft, 70, 109, 173, 175
Witch doctors, 101, 107, 126, 220; *see also* Brujos
Withdrawal, 90, 158
Wizard of the Upper Amazon (Lamb), 101
Women, 12, 20, 113, 168–69, 179, 192
Wounded Knee massacre, 234
Wovoka, 234–35
Wysoccan, 172

Xanthines, 17

Yagé, 55, 99–131, 175; *illus.*, 100, 103; preparation of, 116,

127–29; effects of, 121–24
Yagé Letters (Burroughs), 101
Yarumo, 149–50
Yin and yang, 68–69, 70, 71

Yoga, 8, 10, 26, 70, 71, 178, 201, 244, 256, 259
Yogananda, Paramahansa, 25
Yuca, 146, 149, 152

ABOUT THE AUTHOR

Andrew Weil, M.D., is the best-selling author of ten books, including *Spontaneous Healing, Eating Well for Optimum Health, Eight Weeks to Optimum Health* and, forthcoming, *Healthy Aging*. Dr. Weil has degrees in biology and medicine from Harvard University. He has experienced and studied healers and healing systems around the world and has earned an international reputation as an expert on alternative medicine, mind-body interactions, and medical botany. He is Clinical Professor of Medicine and Director of the Program in Integrative Medicine (www.integrative medicine.arizona.edu) at the University of Arizona in Tucson. Dr. Weil also writes a monthly newsletter, *Self-Healing* (www.drweilselfhealing.com) and has a popular Web site, www.drweil.com.

NATURAL HEALTH, NATURAL MEDICINE
The Complete Guide to Wellness and Self-Care for Optimum Health

A comprehensive guide to preventative health maintenance and the foundation for Dr. Andrew Weil's work on maintaining optimum health. *Natural Health, Natural Medicine* is the bible of natural medicine, featuring general diet and nutrition information as well as simple recipes, answers to readers' most pressing questions, a catalog of home remedies, invaluable resources, and hundreds of practical tips.

ISBN 0-618-47903-1

HEALTH AND HEALING
The Philosophy of Integrative Medicine and Optimum Health

Dr. Weil's groundbreaking handbook for people who want to understand the strengths and weaknesses of conventional and alternative medicine, *Health and Healing* presents the full spectrum of alternative healing practices, including holistic medicine, homeopathy, osteopathy, chiropractic, and Chinese medicine and outlines how they differ from conventional approaches. ISBN 0-618-47908-2

FROM CHOCOLATE TO MORPHINE
WITH WINIFRED ROSEN
Everything You Need to Know About Mind-Altering Drugs

The definitive guide to drugs and drug use, now revised and updated to cover drugs made available in the last decade. This enormously popular book is the best and most authoritative resource for unbiased information about how drugs affect the mind and the body. ISBN 0-618-48379-9

THE NATURAL MIND
A Revolutionary Approach to the Drug Problem

Dr. Weil's first book and the philosophical basis for all of his resulting beliefs and tenets on health, healing, and the mind. Now completely revised and updated for the twenty-first century, this is essential reading for anyone interested in Dr. Weil's philosophy of integrative medicine and optimum health. ISBN 0-618-46513-8

THE MARRIAGE OF THE SUN AND MOON
Dispatches from the Frontiers of Consciousness

A collection of essays about Dr. Weil's travels to South America in the early 1970s in search of information on altered states of consciousness, drug use in other cultures, and other matters having to do with the complementarity of mind and body. These experiences laid the foundation of his mission to restore the connection between medicine and nature. ISBN 0-618-47905-8

Made in the USA
Middletown, DE
10 February 2021